PRAISE FOR
BEYOND CHOICE

"*Beyond Choice* expands upon Dr. DeShawn Taylor's works on abortion access and Reproductive Justice, this time in a workbook, allowing the reader to go on a journey to build upon their own understanding of abortion beyond the choice framework. This book is a great read for anyone who wants to deepen their relationship to Reproductive Justice."

— **RENEE BRACEY SHERMAN**,
Co-Author of *Liberating Abortion*

"*Beyond Choice* makes an invaluable contribution to the fight for Reproductive Justice. It is a powerful tool that can move readers beyond the unproductive, angry polarization that characterizes abortion politics at all levels—from kitchen tables to Congress. This is a book for abortion seekers, grassroots and policy activists, medical providers, and journalists. Reframing abortion in the broader justice context is a gift to individual patients, their families, and their communities. Dr. Taylor's deep knowledge and insights come from years spent as an ally, as an abortion provider, and as an advocate for compassionate and comprehensive care."

—**MARLENE GERBER FRIED**,
Hampshire College,
Emerita Professor

"*Beyond Choice* is truly a gift to the reproductive health, rights, and justice movement that will guide readers from theory to action. Dr. DeShawn Taylor is a force for Reproductive Justice and a fierce advocate for her patients and all people seeking reproductive healthcare. She has studied the landscape, knows how we got to this moment of restriction and prohibition, and with *Beyond Choice*, she provides a transformational guide on how to take Reproductive Justice off the shelf and make it a reality."

—PAMELA MERRITT,
Executive Director,
Medical Students for Choice

"As an abortion provider and social justice leader, Dr. DeShawn Taylor powerfully illustrates how to transform Reproductive Justice theory into action. She has created a best practice guide that will be useful not only for the reproductive health, rights, and justice movements, but also for the many other issue areas that intersect with our collective fight for liberation. *Beyond Choice* is essential reading for anyone who cares deeply about social progress and change."

—BRITTANY FONTENO,
President & CEO,
National Abortion Federation

Dr. Deshawn Taylor has brought her tremendous medical experience, and her profound lived experience to Beyond Choice. At a time where we are being confronted by rage, fear, anxiety, and uncertainty, this resource will help people to channel those feelings into something tangible that deepens us in our reproductive justice values and creates real change. It is my hope that this workbook will not just live on a shelf, but instead it will take flight in the deeds and actions of its readers, so that more of us can be transformed in the service of the work.

—KWAJELYN J. JACKSON,
Executive Director,
Feminist Center for Reproductive Liberation

"In this moment when so many of our rights are under attack, people are looking for ways to engage in meaningful activism. This workbook is an invaluable resource for all of us, whether we are new to the Reproductive Justice movement or seasoned activists. Thoughtfully crafted with a warm, personal tone, it equips activists with insights, practical tools, and a deep understanding of the intersections between reproductive rights, social justice, and systemic change. Its inclusive, intersectional approach provides both clarity and inspiration, making it a must-have for those dedicated to becoming more active in the work of moving toward Reproductive Justice."

—**SUSAN YANOW**, MSW,
Consultant and Activist

"At a time in which women's rights continue to be eroded at an alarming rate, there could be no more urgent moment for a work such as this. This book is the revolutionary roadmap needed to effectively fight back even in the face of life-threatening rights retrenchments and ultimately work towards achieving the goal of Reproductive Justice in America. With the practical tools, case studies, and exercises included herein, there is no longer any excuse to merely sit on the sidelines. The prescription has been written. Now it's up to us to initiate the remedy."

—**AVIS JONES-DEWEEVER**, Ph.D.,
Principal, Nouveaux Strategies

BEYOND CHOICE

An Essential Workbook for Personal and
Community Transformation Through Reproductive Justice

DESHAWN TAYLOR, MD

© **2025 by DeShawn Taylor, MD**
All rights reserved. No part of this book may be reproduced in any form or by any means without written permission from the publisher, except in the case of brief quotations in reviews and critical articles.

Published by Health Justice Press An imprint of Health Justice MD Phoenix, Arizona
Health Justice MD is a registered trademark.
For information, permissions, or other inquiries, please contact: info@healthjusticemd.net.

HEALTH JUSTICE MD

Published January 20, 2026
Printed in the United States of America

ISBN: 979-8-9943341-0-2 (Paperback)
ISBN: 979-8-9943341-1-9 (E-Book)

This book is provided for informational purposes only and does not constitute medical advice, diagnosis, or treatment. Although the author is a licensed physician, the content is not intended as a substitute for professional medical consultation or care. Always seek the advice of a qualified health provider with any questions you may have regarding a medical condition or healthcare decision.

Some names and identifying details have been changed to protect individuals' privacy. The views expressed in this book are those of the author and may not reflect those of her professional affiliations or employers.

Use of the information in this book is at your own risk. Neither the author nor the publisher is responsible for any adverse effects, outcomes, or consequences resulting from the use or application of any of the information provided herein.

Given the rapidly evolving legal, medical, and regulatory landscape surrounding reproductive health and abortion care, readers should verify any laws, clinical guidelines, or policies referenced in this book against current, authoritative sources. Laws vary by jurisdiction and may change at any time.

Health Justice Press is dedicated to amplifying the intersections of medicine and social equity. By bridging clinical expertise with social justice, we publish transformative works that challenge systemic barriers, advocate for reproductive freedom, and empower clinicians, advocates, and communities to build a more just and inclusive healthcare system.

DEDICATION

This work is dedicated to the Reproductive Justice Movement for showing me how to practice medicine with justice at the center, how to train the next generation of providers to acknowledge power dynamics and use their privilege to advocate for the most vulnerable, and how to approach advocacy not as a single issue, but as a holistic pursuit of collective liberation. To the founding Black women and countless visionaries who moved the work forward, your scholarship, activism, and relentless commitment to dignity, autonomy, and intersectional truth-telling did not just shift policy—it fundamentally redefined my professional life. Thank you for the blueprint.

CONTENTS

Introduction: Your Reproductive Justice Journey Begins 11

1 EXAMINING YOUR PERSONAL EXPERIENCE WITH REPRODUCTIVE JUSTICE
In what ways have you participated in oppressive institutional policies and practices related to healthcare? 17

Case Study: When Life Begins (and Ends): The Adriana Smith Story 34

2 MOVING BEYOND "CHOICE"
Which of the tenets of Reproductive Justice most aligns with the work you do or the policies you champion? 45

3 HOW REPRODUCTIVE JUSTICE TOUCHES EVERYTHING
In what ways does Reproductive Justice intersect with other aspects of your life and community? 63

4 CONNECTING THE PERSONAL TO THE POLITICAL
Do you connect the personal to the political? 81

Case Study: The Criminalization of Pregnancy Loss: The Brittany Watts Story ... 109

5 FAITH AND ABORTION CARE
Is there a place for faith in abortion care? 125

6 CULTURE, POWER, AND THE FIGHT FOR INCLUSIVE CARE
Who has access to safe, affirming healthcare, and who is denied it? 145

7 KEEPING THE MOVEMENT ALIVE
How will you sustain your commitment to Reproductive Justice for yourself, your community, and the generations to come? 165

Conclusion: The Work Is Now 189

Notes 193

Resources and Further Reading 199

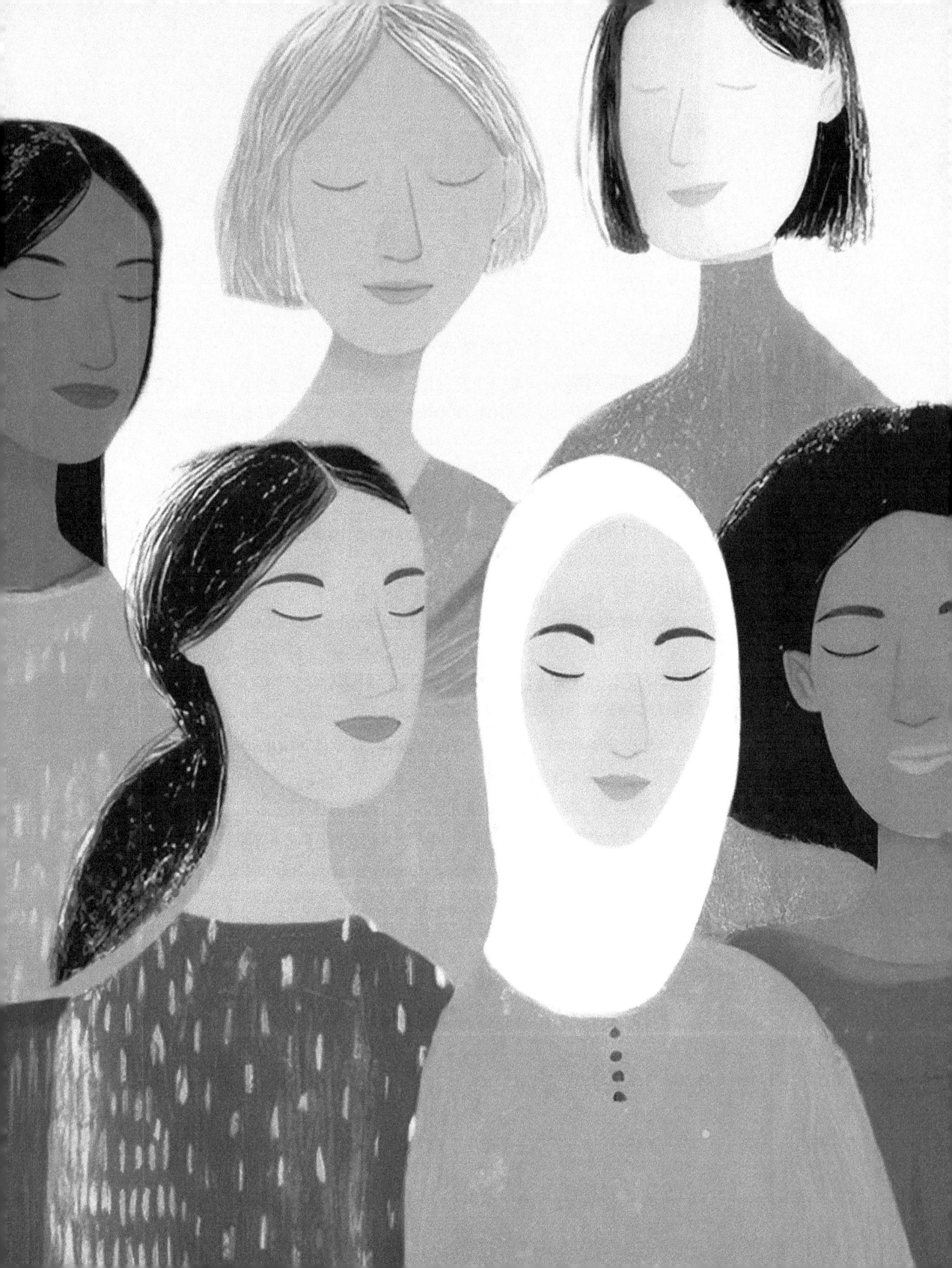

INTRODUCTION

YOUR REPRODUCTIVE JUSTICE JOURNEY BEGINS

In 2022, I wrote *Undue Burden: A Black Woman Physician on Being Christian and Pro-Abortion in the Reproductive Justice Movement.* The US Supreme Court had recently heard the oral arguments for the Dobbs v. Jackson Women's Health Organization case that would ultimately overturn *Roe v. Wade* and upend almost fifty years of legal protections for abortion care in our country. Writing the book during the fall of Roe was a very important outlet for me. As I grappled with the chaos and confusion, I suffered the moral injury of having to turn patients away because the legality, and the perception of legality, of abortion changed daily. Arizona enforced a nineteenth-century abortion ban for a time. It had one narrow exception, to save the life of the pregnant person. In practice, health and life exceptions to bans have often proven to be unworkable, except in the most extreme circumstances, and generally prevent physicians from practicing evidence-based medicine. *Undue Burden* marked the moment and was my offering toward a better future beyond Roe. True liberation requires more than the status quo that was Roe.

After the book was published, I met countless readers at conferences, workshops, and speaking engagements, each with dog-eared, sticky-noted, underlined copies, their thoughts scribbled in the margins. I thought, *My words have touched something deep.*

I also thought, *Those readers' thoughts don't belong in the margins; they belong front and center.*

I wrote this workbook to help people process beyond the margins and hopefully inspire crucial conversations.

Conversations with a text turn into conversations with loved ones, and eventually, conversations lead to action. This is how change happens, one conversation at a time. Readers have told me that they passed their copies of *Undue Burden* on to loved ones who were not sympathetic to the pro-abortion movement. The book helped bridge a divide, laying a foundation for discussions they had long given up on having. Readers who believed that abortion was problematic, often due to religious or other taught values, began to see the complexity of reproductive healthcare in a new way.

What moves me about these stories is that they represent the ripple effect of honest, open dialogue. I've created this workbook to make space for more of these conversations. It provides a space to bring your voice forward and deepen your understanding of yourself, your values, and your communities through the lens of Reproductive Justice.

Your voice is more powerful than you know. Each of us has a role in creating the world in which we want to live, and this workbook will help you discover and shape yours, no matter your background or how actively you want to engage. This workbook is for readers who are:

- Unsure where they stand and just want to learn and explore in a safe, quiet, supportive space.
- Allies of the movement, with a clear vision often expressed through private conversations, donations, occasional letters to lawmakers, social media posts, or petitions.
- Advocates who speak publicly, educate others, attend rallies, fundraise, and join groups.
- Activists who stand shoulder to shoulder with directly impacted individuals, organizing, mobilizing, and maintaining sustained engagement, even putting themselves on the line.

These roles aren't fixed, and most people shift between what they're willing and able to do at different times in their lives—I know I have. This is fine. The movement needs people at all levels. There are many ways to engage with Reproductive Justice work, and all are valid and necessary, whether you're lending a book to a loved one, helping out at your neighborhood abortion clinic, or speaking before your state legislature. We all come to this movement from different backgrounds, with different experiences, knowledge, and resources.

What matters is recognizing and engaging where you are, with your skills, passions, resources, and capacity. This workbook will help you pinpoint ways to do just that.

My journey illustrates how we can keep learning, engaging, and changing. I began as an ally and advocate, focusing on my role as a physician dedicated to providing fair, respectful, patient-centered healthcare. In 2013, I founded Desert Star Family Planning LLC to serve ethnically diverse, medically underserved, and economically depressed communities in Arizona. Desert Star, one of fewer than ten independent abortion clinics owned by an African American in the United States, opened during a period when abortion access in Arizona was rapidly shrinking because of the enactment of laws restricting abortion year after year. Despite these restrictions, *Roe v. Wade* provided a legal baseline across the country, giving us the opportunity to fight to maintain access to abortion care in the state.

There was a point when I became very frustrated with having to comply with a new abortion restriction every year and decided to look into what was happening during the legislative session. Imagine how shocked I was to learn that several anti-abortion bills were introduced every session. Advocates fought hard to keep them from passing through the committees, and usually, only one bad bill made it out of the session. Advocates were victorious in stopping many more bills, but it still felt hollow when any anti-abortion bill was signed into law.

Safe, equitable access to abortion without shame, stigma, or fear of criminalization cannot be achieved without eliminating racial and economic disparities in reproductive health. White supremacy and systemic racism have created and upheld the conditions of unequal access to resources to survive and thrive for Black and Indigenous people of color (BIPOC) and other marginalized communities in the United States. Arizona appeared promising on paper before *Roe v. Wade*. However, the web of restrictions in the law books made abortion care inaccessible for many. Where was the justice in that? For me, seeking Reproductive Justice in Arizona motivated my involvement in activism.

Over the years, I have become an activist, amplifying the voices of those whose stories I carry as a provider and speaking out for myself and my colleagues who are asked to work within an unjust system. My journey from ally to activist has been transformative. I hope your journey, wherever it takes you, will be just as meaningful.

How to Use This Workbook

This workbook aims to clarify concepts beyond the jargon, translating abstract ideas into tangible realities you can recognize in your daily life. It's designed to help you analyze these concepts and place them in the context of your own life. The exercises will prompt you to explore not just what you think, but why you think it, and how those thoughts can lead to meaningful action.

Each chapter is structured to encourage both reflection and action.

1. An opening, thought-provoking question prompts you to examine your existing beliefs and assumptions.
2. Exercises help you explore how family, community, culture, or society has shaped your current values.
3. New ideas—the principles of Reproductive Justice—are introduced. These may create friction with your current beliefs, challenging you to think differently.
4. Additional exercises let you explore your beliefs through this new lens.
5. Goal setting and practical steps are presented that you can incorporate into your life and work.

This workbook encourages you to actively engage with the material, yourself, and your community. The exercises are designed to be challenging, to make you uncomfortable at times, and to push you beyond your comfort zone.

I have always found, for myself, that beyond my comfort zone is where growth happens.

Creating Safe Spaces for Dialogue

While you can work through this book on your own, I encourage you to gather with others to discuss these ideas and exercises.

Here are some suggestions for creating productive discussion spaces:

- **Establish ground rules.** Begin by agreeing on basic guidelines for respectful communication, such as allowing each person to speak without interruption, using "I" statements, and avoiding judgment of others' experiences.

- **Center marginalized voices.** Create space for those most affected by reproductive injustice to share their experiences and perspectives.
- **Practice active listening.** Focus on understanding others rather than formulating your response while they're speaking.
- **Embrace discomfort.** Growth happens when we push beyond what feels comfortable and familiar.
- **Commit to confidentiality.** What's shared in the group stays in the group.
- **Take breaks when needed.** These topics can be emotionally challenging. It's okay to step back and take care of yourself.

This workbook invites you to examine your personal experiences with healthcare systems, reproductive choices, and systemic oppression. This reflection is essential for understanding how we can create change, but it can also bring up difficult emotions and memories. You might notice strong feelings, physical responses, or resistance to certain exercises. All of these responses are normal and deserve respect.

Take care of yourself as you work through this material. Pace yourself, skip exercises that feel overwhelming, and seek support from trusted friends or mental health professionals when needed. If this work brings up memories of serious trauma or medical violence, consider speaking with a counselor familiar with reproductive trauma. Remember that your healing matters, and taking care of yourself as you do this work is wisdom, not weakness. Trust yourself to know what you can handle.

Transformation doesn't happen overnight. This work is ongoing, and each step you take, no matter how small, contributes to the larger movement for Reproductive Justice. As you write in this book, you are essentially creating your own story, with your own insights and experiences. This is a powerful act, and it becomes even more impactful when you take what you've created out into the world to help change lives.

As I wrote in the introduction to *Undue Burden* three years ago:

My vision for this book is realized when those who need reproductive healthcare, those who love and care for them, and those who provide care come together to acknowledge that our oppressions are interconnected. Only then can we center the real-life experiences of people impacted by harmful policies and work together to create better lives, healthier families, and sustainable communities.

This workbook is your invitation to join me in building that world.
Let's get started.

—**DR. DESHAWN TAYLOR**,
December 1, 2025

CHAPTER 1

EXAMINING YOUR PERSONAL EXPERIENCE WITH REPRODUCTIVE JUSTICE

> In what ways have you participated in oppressive institutional policies and practices related to healthcare?

Why This Question?

Mapping your personal journey through the healthcare system is important. Why? First, speaking about your experience helps you understand what changes are necessary for you personally. You can't initiate change unless you know exactly what change you want to see, whether you're a medical professional, a patient, a loved one of someone seeking care, or even a concerned bystander.

Second, acknowledging your personal journey through the healthcare system allows you to connect your experience to a bigger picture. When you see that bigger picture, you start to understand that you're not alone and that change can happen if everyone affected by the same issues works together.

In that spirit of open hearts and collective action, let's turn inward and examine your personal experience.

In what ways have you participated in oppressive institutional policies and practices related to healthcare?

I have been harmed by an oppressive healthcare institution when…

I have harmed someone else by my role in an oppressive healthcare institution when….

Was remembering your own oppression easier than thinking of a time you played a role in someone else's oppression?

_____
_____
_____
_____
_____
_____

Our Shared Experience

In my experience, most people readily identify how healthcare systems have harmed them but struggle to recognize how they might be contributing to harm. This is natural. We're taught to see ourselves as individuals navigating systems, not as participants in those systems.

For example, when I ask people during workshops to reflect on how they have participated in oppressive policies or institutions, the following are some responses I often hear.

How People Feel Harmed (Common)
- "My doctor dismissed my pain during pregnancy."
- "I couldn't get an appointment when I needed one."
- "The forms didn't have options that fit my family structure."
- "I was judged for my choices about having children."
- "I couldn't afford the care I needed."

How People Acknowledge Causing Harm (Much Less Common)
- "I stayed silent when a colleague made an inappropriate comment."
- "I didn't question a policy that excluded certain patients."
- "I've judged others for their reproductive choices."
- "I've repeated harmful myths about certain types of patients."
- "I withheld information from my doctor because I thought he would judge me."

Think about the examples above. Did any of them remind you of your own experiences? If so, add your recollections:

_____
_____
_____
_____
_____
_____

Our Shared Values

We often cause or accept harm because of deeply ingrained values we learned growing up—values we may not even realize we've internalized. Do you recognize any of the values listed below in yourself?

Values I Hold/Values I Don't Hold

My Values	YES, I Hold This Value	NO, I Don't Hold This Value	Unsure
Obedience to authority			
Privacy above all			
Personal responsibility for experiences			
Compliance with systems			
Don't speak up—it's not your place			
Trust professionals without question			
Stay neutral to avoid conflict			
Avoid discussing taboo topics (e.g., abortion, sexuality)			
Put others' needs above your own			
Acceptance of "That's just how things are"			
Defer to those with more experience			
Focus on individual merit			
Keep emotions out of decision-making			
Stay loyal to family or community norms			
Health is just a personal issue			
If it doesn't affect me, it's not my concern			

Did any of these values influence your actions or decisions when you participated in the oppressive healthcare situations you described above? For example:

- Were you taught to "not question doctors"?
- Did you believe it was "not your place" to speak up?
- Were you trying to "follow the rules" without considering the broader consequences?

Space for reflection: _____
_____
_____
_____
_____
_____

Where do you think these values came from?
- Family teachings?
- Cultural or community expectations?
- Religious beliefs?
- Messages from media, school, or institutions?
- All or none of the above?

Space for reflection: _____
_____
_____
_____
_____
_____

New Thinking: Understanding Privilege and Power in the Healthcare Setting

We all carry values and beliefs about reproduction, family, healthcare, and autonomy that were instilled in us long before we could examine them critically. These beliefs often operate below our conscious awareness, yet they shape how we interact with healthcare systems and with each other.

Many of us hold onto these values without realizing that they were shaped by incomplete information or societal norms. We gain an opportunity to grow when we are presented with new perspectives, especially ones that challenge our comfort zones. We all need to constantly examine and rethink what we thought we knew about healthcare, oppression, and personal responsibility. These issues aren't simple. But when we clearly know our values and why we hold them, we are able to better exercise our privilege and power instead of giving that power away to unexamined beliefs.

Once we understand our power, we can create change. When we think about dismantling an institutional practice like healthcare, we often see it as a massive, impenetrable structure. This isn't true. The healthcare system is made up of institutions, and institutions are made up of people.

Change happens when we influence the people who make up institutions. However, the first person we must change is ourselves.

We must determine what we need from a system and then figure out how to reach the individuals within that system who have the power.

Dismantling oppressive systems requires understanding how institutions function.

People within institutions often create policies that don't affect them personally. If they did, they might not support them. People outside of institutions who interact with bad policy can unwittingly contribute to their oppression by being passive. Patients, practitioners, community members, family members, and friends all have a role to play in how we experience reproductive healthcare.

DID YOU KNOW?

Oppressive systems: Policies, practices, and institutions that consistently limit some people's access to resources or dignity while benefiting others. In healthcare, this includes insurance exclusions, discriminatory protocols, or research that ignores certain populations.

Complicity: Participating in or going along with harmful systems, often without realizing it. We're all complicit in various systems because we live within them. Recognizing this helps us choose different actions.

Privilege: Unearned advantages based on identity or circumstances. In healthcare, this might mean having insurance, speaking your doctor's language, or being believed when reporting symptoms. Having privilege doesn't mean your life is easy; it means certain barriers don't affect you.

My Story

My experiences as an ob-gyn and an abortion provider reveal some of the values that led me to be an unintentional participant in an oppressive system. It's important to remember that our participation doesn't make us bad people; it makes us human beings shaped by our culture and context.

For example, I worked at a hospital where pregnant incarcerated women were shackled to their beds during labor. When I questioned this practice, I was told it was policy. For too long, I accepted this answer without challenging it. Eventually, I gathered the conviction to challenge this policy. I recall telling the officer, "Where is she going to go? She's in labor." That day, I learned that the guards could practice discretion and remove the shackles. And that I was complicit in a system that was dehumanizing women at their most vulnerable when I didn't question the policy or the officer.

Another example of my complicity in an oppressive healthcare system happened when I participated in a C-section on a woman who refused the procedure. There was a hospital policy that two doctors could sign off that the procedure was medically necessary, allowing it to proceed without the patient's consent. My participation in overriding her bodily autonomy—even to save her baby—has stayed with me for decades. I was complicit in a traumatic experience that stemmed from a system valuing the potential life inside her over her own autonomy, and yet, I would make the same choice today. The role of an obstetrician once a pregnant person goes into labor is to deliver a healthy baby while preserving the health of the person birthing the baby. These issues aren't simple! Sometimes, each available option to choose causes someone harm. There isn't always a safe answer.

A Shift in Thinking: From Passive to Active

Remember the list of values from earlier? Here are some examples of how to reframe them.

Original (Passive) Values	Emerging (Active) Values
Obedience to authority	Critical thinking and accountability to community
Privacy above all	Transparency and informed communication
Personal responsibility only	Collective responsibility and community care
Compliance with systems	Advocacy for systemic change
Don't speak up—it's not your place	Speak up and advocate for yourself and others
Trust professionals without question	Informed consent and shared decision-making
Stay neutral to avoid conflict	Engage in constructive confrontation for justice
Avoid discussing taboo topics (e.g., abortion, sexuality)	Normalize open dialogue on difficult issues
Put others' needs above your own	Balance personal boundaries with compassion
Acceptance of the status quo	Belief in the possibility of change
Defer to those with more experience	Value lived experience and diverse perspectives
Focus on individual merit	Recognize systemic barriers and privilege
Keep emotions out of decision-making	Integrate emotions with rational thought
Stay loyal to family or community norms	Cultivate personal values while honoring roots
Health is just a personal issue	Understand health as a societal and collective issue
If it doesn't affect me, it's not my concern	Practice empathy and allyship for others' struggles

Discuss your reflections with a trusted friend, family member, or community group. What would you tell them about your participation in the healthcare system now that you've seen your role differently? Organize your thoughts here using these prompts:

- "I used to believe ____, but now I believe ____."
- "I never realized how much ____ influenced my thinking until now."
- "I was taught ____, but after thinking deeply, I see things differently because ____."
- "Moving forward, I want to focus on ____ because ____."

Example:

- I used to believe that staying quiet was respectful, but now I believe that it's my responsibility to speak up to prevent harm.
- I was taught to trust authority figures no matter what, but now I understand that questioning them can lead to better outcomes.

From Thinking to Action: Finding Your Voice

Transformation is incomplete without action. Articulating your new values solidifies your understanding and empowers you to advocate for yourself and others. This section will help you find words that reflect your changed beliefs and explore how to apply them in real-life situations.

Reflection Questions

Personal Experience: Now that you've read this chapter, have you thought of any more times that you've participated in oppressive institutional policies or practices related to healthcare?

_____
_____
_____
_____
_____
_____

Emotional Response: How did the information in this chapter make you feel? More vulnerable or more powerful? _____

_____
_____
_____
_____
_____

Knowledge and Skills: Do you have any specific skills that might make you a valuable ally or activist? For example, are you a healthcare practitioner, or has your experience given you a story to tell? _____

_____
_____
_____
_____
_____

Community Need: In your community, where does oppression within the healthcare system seem most urgent or overlooked? _____
_____
_____
_____
_____
_____
_____

Existing Movements: Do you know of or are you already involved in other social justice movements that intersect with your experiences within the healthcare system? For example, are you part of a church group or women's group where your stories could be useful, or could you harness these groups to focus on this issue? _____
_____
_____
_____
_____
_____
_____

Personal Values: Which values have been most challenged by the ideas in this chapter? How does that make you feel? _____
_____
_____
_____
_____
_____
_____

Impact Assessment: Where do you believe your contribution could make the greatest difference in challenging oppressive practices in the healthcare system? Consider both the need and your capacity to affect change in that area.

_____
_____
_____
_____
_____
_____

Your Turn

Draft a personal commitment statement summarizing your next steps relating to oppressions in the healthcare system.

You can use this template:

My Commitment:

I recognize that I was taught _____, but through reflection and learning, I now value _____. Moving forward, I will _____ to align my actions with these values. I understand that living this way may be challenging, but I am committed to _____ because I believe in _____.

Example:

I recognize that I was taught to stay silent when I witnessed injustice, but now I value speaking up for myself and others. Moving forward, I will challenge oppressive comments and policies when I encounter them. I know this may be uncomfortable, but I am committed to creating safer environments because I believe everyone deserves dignity and respect.

Imagine situations where you can apply your new values. Write down or role-play how you'd respond differently now:

- A doctor dismisses your concern. How do you advocate for yourself?
- You hear a friend make an insensitive comment about healthcare access. What do you say?
- You encounter a policy at work that feels unjust. How might you challenge it constructively?

Example Scenario:

Old Response: Stay quiet during a rushed doctor's appointment.
New Response: "I understand you're busy, but I need to ensure my concerns are heard. Can we take a moment to discuss this thoroughly?"

Setting Actionable Goals

Based on your reflections, set three concrete actions you'll take to live out your new values. Here are some examples to get you started:

New Value	Action Step	Timeline	Support Needed
Advocacy	Speak up during my next healthcare visit	Next appointment	Practice responses beforehand
Transparency	Share my healthcare experience with a family member or friend	This month	Find a local or online group
Community Care	Volunteer with an organization addressing healthcare disparities	This month	Research local opportunities

If you feel ready, share your story with someone you trust. Speaking your new values out loud can reinforce your transformation. If you prefer privacy, consider writing a letter to yourself to revisit later.

This is how I participated in oppressive institutional policies and practices related to healthcare in the past, and this is what I'm going to change moving forward:

_____
_____
_____
_____

Chapter 1 Summary

As we close this first chapter, take a moment to reflect on the transformative process you've begun. You've examined deeply held values about healthcare and reproductive autonomy, identified how these beliefs shaped your experiences, and encountered new perspectives that challenge traditional thinking about power and personal responsibility.

This work isn't easy. Recognizing our participation in systems that cause harm, even unintentionally, can be uncomfortable. But this discomfort is where growth begins.

Remember that transformation is a continuous journey, not a destination. Be patient with yourself through this process.

In the next chapter, we'll explore how to move beyond the limited "choice" framework to embrace a more comprehensive understanding of Reproductive Justice, connecting your personal experiences to broader political and social contexts.

Room for Thought

CASE STUDY

WHEN LIFE BEGINS (AND ENDS): THE ADRIANA SMITH STORY

> *"It's torture for me. I come here and I see my daughter breathing... but she's not there… It should've been left up to the family."*
> —April Newkirk, Adriana Smith's mother[1]

Adriana Smith, a Black, thirty-year-old nurse and mother from Georgia, was about nine weeks pregnant in February of 2025 when she sought treatment for severe headaches and was sent home with medication. The next morning, her boyfriend found her in distress and called 911. Doctors declared her brain-dead due to blood clots that had formed in her brain. Despite being legally dead, doctors at Emory Medical Center put her on life support, intending to keep her body functioning until the fetus she was carrying reached thirty-two weeks of gestation[2] and could potentially be safely delivered. To achieve this, her body would have to be kept functioning for almost six months.

Smith's situation arose because of a Georgia abortion law known as the Living Infants Fairness and Equality (LIFE) Act, which passed in 2019 but was only enforced after *Roe v. Wade* was overturned in 2022. The law establishes "fetal personhood"—the idea that embryos and fetuses have legal rights. Often called a "heartbeat law," this legislation bans most abortions once fetal cardiac activity is detected, typically around six weeks of pregnancy, before many people have processed the reality that they are pregnant.

What should doctors have done when confronted with potential criminal prosecution due to the LIFE Act?

Georgia Attorney General Chris Carr's office stated, "There is nothing in the LIFE Act that requires medical professionals to keep a woman on life support after brain death. Removing life support is not an action 'with the purpose to terminate a pregnancy.'"[3]

However, Emory Healthcare, the hospital holding Smith's body, stated that it "uses consensus from clinical experts, medical literature, and legal guidance to support our providers as they make individualized treatment recommendations in compliance with Georgia's abortion laws and all other applicable laws."[4] In other words, they felt their hands were tied.

Republican State Senator Edward Setzler, who sponsored Georgia's abortion law, supported the hospital's interpretation: "I think it is completely appropriate that the hospital does what they can to save the life of the child. I think this is an unusual circumstance, but I think it highlights the value of innocent human life."[5]

On June 13, 2025, Adriana's baby, named Chance by his family, was delivered by emergency C-section at just twenty-five weeks, weighing one pound and thirteen ounces. As of late October 2025, he remained in neonatal intensive care. Adriana was removed from life support after the birth and has since been laid to rest after her body was kept "alive" for over four months. Her older son, seven-year-old Chase, is now in counseling as the family navigates their grief. April Newkirk, Adriana's mother, responding to the abortion law, told *The Independent*, "I want them to know that this didn't have to happen…Women have rights; it's their body."[6]

How did you feel when you read Adriana's story?

Take a moment to write down your immediate emotional response: _____

_____
_____
_____
_____
_____
_____

Do you agree with the doctors prioritizing the legal interpretation of "fetal personhood" over established medical consensus regarding brain death and the patient's dignity? Why or why not? _____

_____
_____
_____
_____
_____
_____

If you were in Adriana's situation, what would you want to happen? Is your reasoning dependent on your marital status, your financial status, your religious beliefs, or other factors? _____

_____
_____
_____
_____
_____
_____

If she were further along in her pregnancy, for example, at twenty weeks, would that change how you feel about her situation?

_____
_____
_____
_____
_____
_____

Doctors told the family that the fetus showed signs of potential health complications, including fluid on the brain, which could leave it blind, unable to walk, or even cause it to die during or soon after birth. Does this change your opinion about Adriana and her family's situation? _____

_____
_____
_____
_____
_____
_____

Now that the baby has been delivered by C-section and is in the neonatal intensive care unit, does this change your opinion of what happened? Why or why not? _____

_____
_____
_____
_____
_____
_____

Religious Extremism and the Law

The complexity of the "when life begins" question stems from the tension between biological reality and legal or theological definitions. Biologically, the human reproductive process is highly inefficient: between 30 percent and 50 percent of fertilized eggs never successfully implant, and 15 percent to 20 percent of pregnancies established after implantation end in miscarriage (spontaneous abortion). Given that a significant percentage of conceptions are naturally expelled, the legal move to grant personhood status to a zygote or blastocyst is viewed by many as a concept disconnected from what we scientifically know about human reproduction. As scholar and author Katha Pollitt puts it, the idea that life begins at conception is "an incoherent, covertly religious idea that falls apart if you look at it closely. Few people believe it, as shown by the exceptions they are willing to make."[7]

This complexity is further highlighted by the diverse and evolving perspectives on the beginning of life found across major faith communities, including many Christian denominations:

- Catholics believed for centuries that ensoulment happened forty to ninety days after conception, until the Church revised its position in 1869 to say it occurs at conception.
- Some Jewish traditions consider the fetus part of the mother's body until birth, when the baby takes its first breath.
- Many Muslims believe that ensoulment occurs at 120 days—about six to seven weeks before the fetus is viable outside the womb.[8]

Stories like Adriana's reveal the consequences of enshrining a particular group's religious beliefs about the beginning of life into law.

Should the existence of "life" automatically mean that a zygote's or fetus's life takes precedence over the person's? Or should the life of the pregnant person—and their agency—come first? How should that balance be decided?

What if the survival of the pregnant person is not a matter of life and death, but of illness, injury, or long-term health risks? Does this change your thinking about whose rights should prevail?

Georgia's laws give a fetus "personhood" status. This means that you can claim your fetus as a dependent on your taxes, and harming a fetus can carry the same legal consequences as harming a living person. What are your thoughts on this part of the law?

My Reflections

My practice of medicine is my ministry. Part of that ministry means standing against the weaponization of faith to cause harm. Extremist Christians who proclaim that life begins at conception do not have a monopoly on caring about people's spiritual needs. Fundamentalists don't have the final say on the word of God.

When we allow one narrow religious view to become law, we create situations like Adriana's, where families are robbed of their right to exercise their autonomy, including bodily autonomy and the autonomy to live their beliefs.

When I'm in my clinic and patients want to pray, I take their hand, close my eyes, and meditate until the words come to me, based on whatever is passing between us at that moment. It's completely individual. I work from the idea that God lives within us and that we can tap into Him to guide us. We can do that by meditating or reading the Bible, or whatever someone's ritual and practice is. Whether my patients believe in Christianity, Islam, Judaism—whatever their faith—I'm able to connect. We all share the belief that there is a higher power and that we can access it as individuals, acting on its message.

Uncovering distortions and mistruths from those who use religion as a cloak to gain power and control takes diligence and education. The so-called pro-life movement is highly skilled at manipulating the faithful. I have seen so much damage done in their name throughout my life and practice. Understanding their motives and tactics helps restore faith to its rightful place—inside the heart of each person, within the work of a compassionate society, among caring doctors, and out of our purportedly secular state.

Your Turn

What struck you most about this case?

- ☐ The violation of the family's wishes
- ☐ Worry over who will care for the baby if it survives and who will make that decision
- ☐ The use of a brain-dead person's body without consent
- ☐ The misuse of medical resources and worry over her family's burden of paying for her "care"
- ☐ The trauma to Adriana's living child
- ☐ The precedent this sets for state control over women's bodies
- ☐ The experimental aspect of the situation—keeping a body alive to incubate a fetus for four months is not common medical care
- ☐ The imposition of one faith's religious ideas on everyone
- ☐ The government making medical decisions

From Faith to Action

Do you believe systemic racism played a role in Adriana's death?

Consider this:

Adriana's mother wrote on her GoFundMe page: "Adriana complained about a headache days prior and traveled to two hospitals but was given medication with no tests run or proper examination."[9]

We don't know exactly why Adriana was sent away from the hospital the night before her death, but we do know that for White women, maternal deaths in Georgia are twice the national average, and for Black women, they are six times the national average.[10]

How might viewing her story through a Reproductive Justice lens inspire meaningful action?

Consider the options.

a) Yes, systemic racism likely influenced how Adriana was treated before her death.
   → *Action:* Support Black-led advocacy organizations working to hold hospitals accountable and call your state legislators to demand funding for maternal health equity programs.

b) No, I think her death was more likely due to individual error or plain bad luck.
   → *Action:* Keep your focus on fighting abortion bans like the "heartbeat laws" that made this situation possible. Share how your faith supports bodily autonomy and family rights. When you hear people claim their interpretation is the only valid one, speak up. Advocate for laws that respect families' wishes and religious diversity.

c) I'm not sure. I need to learn more about Adriana's story.
   → *Action:* Read about her story. Discuss it with your friends and loved ones. Journal about it: How would you feel in her situation? Meanwhile, focus on fighting six-week heartbeat laws and other topics you feel strongly about.

Every action is needed, no matter where you stand on the issues. Caring about reproductive rights doesn't require agreeing with every framing, but it does require caring about real impacts.

Further Reflection: The Power of Language

Language has shaped how Adriana's story is told and what people believe about it.

For example, Georgia's LIFE Act bans abortion after cardiac activity is detected, but statutes are written with phrases like "heartbeat," when a "heart" does not, in the traditional way we use the word, exist. Even the term "LIFE" is ironic, as Adriana was brain-dead throughout her ordeal. These choices cloak arbitrary mandates in moral and emotional language.

The media uses its own euphemisms. *People* magazine, along with many other outlets, wrote that Adriana was "kept alive until she delivered her baby" and that she "gave birth."[11] But Adriana was not alive—she had been declared brain-dead in February. And the words "delivered" and "gave birth" suggest agency, as though she labored or participated in the birth. In reality, she underwent a surgical procedure while legally deceased. These word choices blur the line between medical fact and cultural storytelling, shaping readers' sympathies without fully acknowledging the strangeness of keeping a brain-dead body functioning for four months, then cutting a baby, just over one pound, out of it.

How does language like "heartbeat bill," "kept alive," or "gave birth" influence your emotional response to the story?

What is lost, or gained, when euphemisms soften the reality of what happened to Adriana and her family?

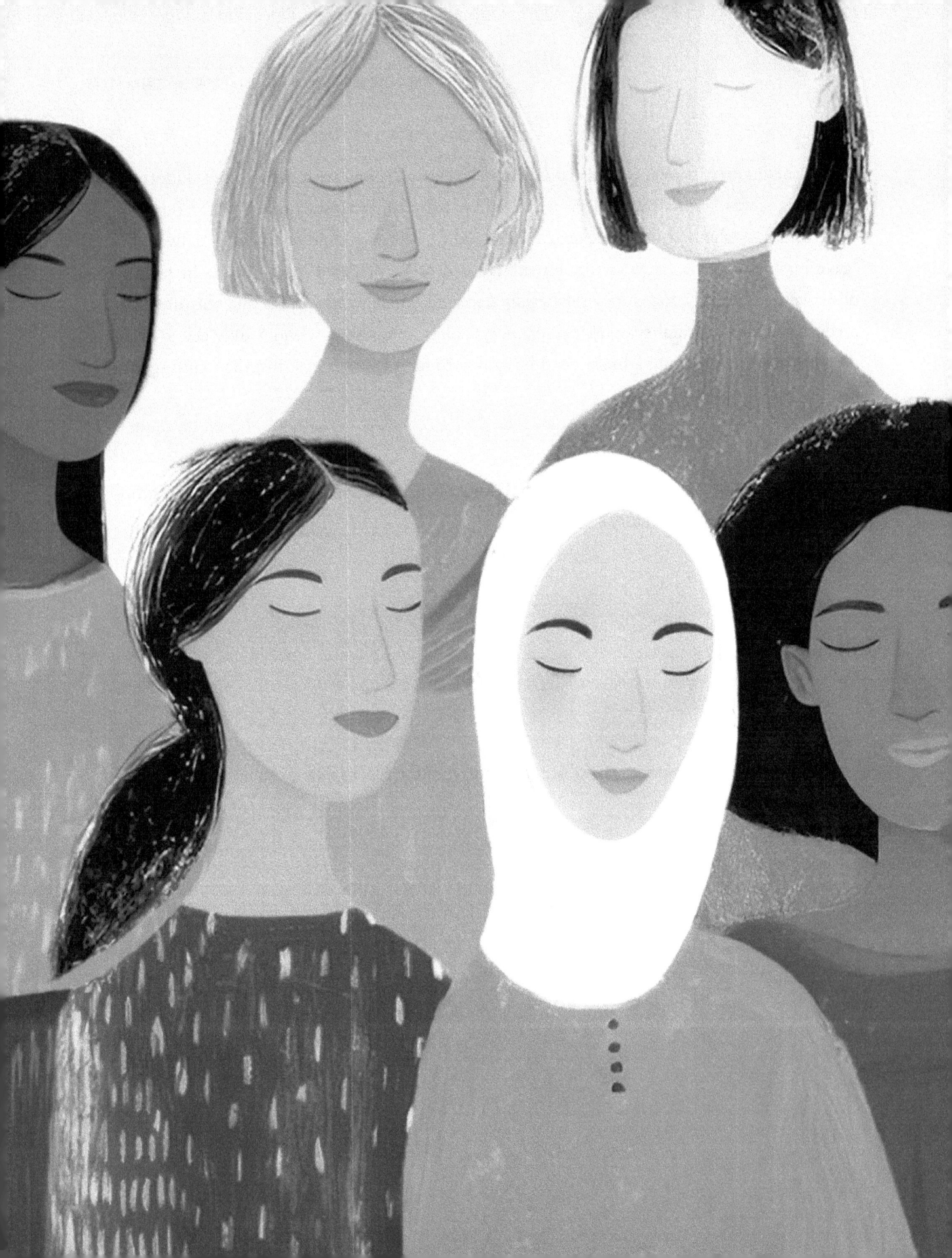

CHAPTER 2

MOVING BEYOND "CHOICE"

> Which tenet of Reproductive Justice most aligns with the work you do or the policies you champion?

Why This Question?

By recognizing which aspects of Reproductive Justice speak most to your values and experiences, you can focus your energy where it will have the greatest impact.

If you don't know the four tenets of Reproductive Justice, don't worry, that's what this chapter is about. First, though, we'll unpack the limitations of the "choice" framework that has dominated reproductive rights conversations for decades. We do this because it's important to understand how we've been taught to think and talk about reproductive care before we can undo that thinking and create a new language and set of values.

This new conversation will help you pinpoint your passions and find your lane for meaningful action: moving beyond "choice."

Our Shared Experience

Most people understand reproductive rights solely through the lens of being pro-choice or pro-life. This narrow perspective can prevent us from seeing the full complexity of reproductive health decisions and the many factors that influence them.

For example, when I ask people about their stance on reproductive rights during workshops and in my clinical practice, I hear some common responses that I call the "but" phrases:

- "I'm pro-choice, but I wouldn't have an abortion myself."
- "I believe in choice, but people shouldn't use abortion as birth control."
- "I'm pro-choice, but why not just have the baby and place it for adoption?"
- "I'm pro-choice, but I think there should be some restrictions."
- "I'm pro-choice, but multiple abortions are a sticking point with me."

Are there times you've caught yourself saying "I support choice, but..." that aren't listed above? What would you add to this list? _____

_____
_____
_____
_____
_____

If you agree with any of the above statements, can you explain why? For example, "I'm pro-choice, but I think there should be some restrictions because…."

_____
_____
_____
_____
_____

If you didn't agree with any of the above statements, can you explain why? For example, "I'm pro-choice and I think there should not be any restrictions on abortion because…."

_____
_____
_____
_____
_____

Question for Thought

Looking at your statements above, do you think there are ways your beliefs about choice are shaped by your own privileges or the lack of them?

_____
_____
_____
_____
_____

Our Shared Values

These "but" statements expose what author Katha Pollitt, in her book *Pro,* calls the "muddled middle." These are "millions of Americans who don't want to ban abortion exactly, but don't want it to be widely available either." It's an attitude of "permit but discourage." They accept the narrative that there is "grief, shame, and stigma" in ending their pregnancies, while also claiming that it's just fine for others. In other words, Pollitt explains, they believe, "You can have your abortion as long as you feel really, really bad about it."[12]

Professor and activist Marlene Fried explains the limits of this kind of thinking, which grows out of the "choice" framework:

1. Choice sets up a simple for/against divide. Reproductive issues are more complex, involving multiple human rights issues.
2. Choice is about the right not to have a child, but it ignores eugenics, population control, and the right to parent in safe communities. That is, many people are fighting for the right to *have* and safely raise children.
3. Choice was framed as anti-government ("Keep the government out of our wombs!") in order to appeal to conservatives. Justice demands the involvement of the government ("Fund universal daycare!").
4. Choice didn't solve the problems of capitalism. If you didn't have money, you really didn't have a choice in America's privatized medical system.
5. Choice is about individuals. It ignores community and social barriers that prevent people from accessing their rights.
6. Choice is about people who have privilege, not the marginalized or oppressed.
7. Choice is not a powerful moral argument in the face of "life."
8. Choice is not a compelling enough vision to sustain an activist, grassroots movement.[13]

The mainstream women's movement of the 1970s that brought us Roe was focused on the concerns of middle-class, cisgender women. It was framed as pro-choice because this type of woman had a choice: she could stay home with her children or not. She could access abortion care or not. Meanwhile, millions of people found themselves in situations without any choice at all. They had to work to survive, so staying home to raise children wasn't really ever a choice. Abortion care often wasn't a choice either because of ever-growing restrictions and lack of resources that put access out of reach.

Which of Fried's limitations of the "choice" framework resonates most with you? Why?

_____
_____
_____
_____
_____
_____

Have you ever felt that the "choice" framework inadequately captured your experience or values? How so?

_____
_____
_____
_____
_____
_____

New Thinking: Understanding Reproductive Justice

The term "Reproductive Justice" was coined in 1994 by a group of American Black women in Chicago who founded Women of African Descent for Reproductive Justice. The four main tenets of Reproductive Justice are:

1. The right to bodily autonomy.
2. The right to have children.
3. The right to not have children.
4. The right to nurture the children we have in a safe and healthy environment.

While mainstream, mostly White, feminist groups continued to focus on choice, groups like the National Black Feminist Organization, the Third World Women's Alliance, and the Committee for Abortion Rights and Against Sterilization Abuse were focusing on these wider issues. They tried to talk about the Hyde Amendment—which bans the use of federal funds for abortion care—forced sterilization, unsafe neighborhoods, and how their struggles intersected with human rights struggles around the world, but their interests were treated as secondary at best.

Three years later, in 1997, SisterSong was founded. This collective, led by sixteen separate POC-headed organizations, came together to support reproductive health for women of color. It included Native American, African American, Latine, and Asian American leadership. Loretta Ross, a co-founder of SisterSong, explained the need for the new movement: "Reducing women's lives down to just whether or not choice is available, we felt was inadequate...choice and abortion... that's all they wanted to talk about."[14]

As activist Loretta Ross wrote:

> *...the ability of any woman to determine her own reproductive destiny is directly linked to the conditions in her community, and these conditions are not just a matter of individual choice and access. For example, a woman cannot make an individual decision about her body if she is part of a community whose human rights as a group are violated, such as through environmental dangers or insufficient quality health care.*[15]

Reproductive Justice is an intersectional theory. It focuses on how the ability to determine one's own reproductive destiny is linked directly to the conditions of one's community. These conditions are not a matter of individual choice and access. They are not about a person's demand for privacy or bodily autonomy. Instead, Reproductive Justice focuses on the social forces that are outside of a person's individual control. It takes the blame and responsibility off the individual and puts it squarely where it belongs: on society and its values.

DID YOU KNOW?

Intersectional theory is a way of understanding that people's identities are never just one thing, but a unique blend of characteristics such as race, gender, class, and ability. It teaches us that these intersecting identities create distinct experiences of privilege and oppression. For instance, while a White, wealthy, straight, able-bodied woman with American citizenship and a White, wealthy, queer, able-bodied woman with American citizenship both face sexism, the challenges and biases they encounter will be fundamentally different due to the added layer of homophobia impacting the queer woman.

Reproductive Justice uses this thinking because when someone is making decisions about having kids, everything in their life matters—their race, how much money they have, where they live, their immigration status, and so on. That's why Reproductive Justice talks about childcare and safe neighborhoods, not just abortion access.

The Four Pillars of Reproductive Justice

Let's look at the four pillars of the Reproductive Justice framework more closely:

1. **The right to bodily autonomy:** Every person should have control over what happens to their body, including reproductive decisions, without coercion or force.
2. **The right to have children:** People should be able to choose to have children regardless of their circumstances, identity, or socioeconomic status.
3. **The right to not have children:** People should have access to contraception, comprehensive sex education, and abortion care regardless of their location, income, or identity.
4. **The right to parent children in safe and sustainable communities:** People who choose to have children should have the resources and support to raise them in healthy, safe environments.

These rights were never a reality for many people, especially those without economic resources and people of color.

Reflection Exercise

Rank the four pillars of Reproductive Justice from most to least resonant with your personal values or work: _____

1. _____

2. _____

3. _____

4. _____

What makes your top-ranked pillar particularly meaningful to you? _____

_____
_____
_____
_____
_____
_____

Let's go back to the question that opened this chapter: **Which tenet of Reproductive Justice most aligns with the work you do or the policies you champion?**

Can you rephrase your work or passions in the language and framework of Reproductive Justice? _____

_____
_____
_____
_____
_____
_____

My Story

As a physician and Reproductive Justice advocate, the tenet that resonates most deeply with me is the right to parent children in safe and sustainable communities.

People are often surprised when I say this because they see me solely as an abortion provider. They assume that the most important tenet to me must be the right not to have a child. In fact, it's ironic: that tenet ranks fourth for me, not because it's least unimportant, but because my work and lived experience have shown me how deeply unjust the world can be for those who *do* want to raise families—particularly Black and Brown families, poor families, queer families, and undocumented families.

Many of the people who come to me for abortion care already have children. They are in my clinic because they are struggling to raise those families in safe environments.

The right to parent with dignity, support, and freedom from surveillance or violence is too often denied. That is the injustice that most haunts me—and most motivates me.

When I founded Desert Star Family Planning Clinic, I wasn't just opening a medical facility. I was creating a space where marginalized communities could receive dignified, culturally competent care. I've seen firsthand how the system fails Black mothers, how poverty is criminalized, and how families are torn apart not because parents don't love their children, but because they lack resources and support. Now, my clinic has evolved into the nonprofit Health Justice Clinic, where we don't just deliver healthcare; we address people's lives before and after they leave our clinic.

The right to parent children in safe and sustainable communities is central to everything I do. When I train medical students and residents, I teach them to look beyond the immediate medical concern to see the whole person, including their transportation challenges, childcare needs, financial constraints, and community context. I tell them, "To really make a patient's life better, doctors must also address and advocate to improve the conditions that impact a patient's decision to start or add to their families at a given moment in time."

When I advocate at the state legislature, I fight against bills that criminalize pregnancy outcomes and push for policies that support families. I've seen how in Arizona, funds meant to help poor families are instead used to investigate them and place their children in foster care. By doing this, the state is saying that people with low income do not have the right to be parents, especially if they're Black, and that is something that I cannot stand for.

My commitment to this tenet led me to establish Desert Star Institute for Family Planning, a nonprofit that complements my clinic's services. We've expanded beyond abortion training to provide long-term contraceptives to uninsured people, provide community education, and engage in policy advocacy. We understand that reproductive health doesn't exist in isolation—it's connected to housing, education, economic opportunity, and freedom from violence.

By centering this pillar of Reproductive Justice in my work, I've found a more powerful way to fight for reproductive freedom than focusing on abortion access alone. It has allowed me to build coalitions with others working on racial justice, economic justice, and healthcare equity. It reminds me daily that my practice is my ministry—a place where spirituality meets social justice in service of creating communities where all families can thrive.

A Shift in Thinking: From Choice to Justice

As we move from a "choice" framework to a Reproductive Justice framework, we need to transform how we think about reproductive healthcare. Here are some ways our values might shift:

"Choice" Values	Reproductive Justice Values
Individual right to privacy	Collective human rights and community well-being
Focus on abortion access only	Focus on the full spectrum of reproductive needs, including resources needed to raise a family
Emphasis on legal rights	Emphasis on access and resources
"My body, my choice."	"Our bodies, our communities, our futures."
Abortion as a personal decision	View healthcare within a social context
Government shouldn't interfere	Government should provide support and resources
Politically neutral	Explicitly political and intersectional
Centered on privileged women	Centered on the most marginalized
Single-issue advocacy	Engagement in multi-issue movement building

Reflection Exercise

Which value from the right side of the chart above challenges or surprises you the most? Why do you think this is?

_____
_____
_____
_____
_____
_____

Which shift in values from the left to the right chart excites you the most? Why?

_____
_____
_____
_____
_____
_____
_____

From Thinking to Action: Reproductive Justice in Action

When we apply Reproductive Justice principles to our work, it transforms how we engage with healthcare systems, communities, and policymaking:

- **In healthcare settings**, we see ourselves and others as whole people impacted by social contexts, not just individual medical cases. We consider transportation barriers, financial constraints, family responsibilities, and culture when seeking, providing, or supporting others in accessing care.
- **In community organizing**, we build coalitions across issues like housing, economic justice, racial equity, LGBTQIA rights, and environmental justice, recognizing how they all impact reproductive autonomy.

- **In policy advocacy**, we push for comprehensive solutions beyond abortion access, including paid family leave, affordable childcare, universal healthcare, living wages, and educational opportunities.

When we focus on communities, we focus on raising up the traditional wisdom that resides within communities.

In moving beyond Roe to something that works for everyone, we must center the most marginalized, impacted people and their communities in a way that helps and engages them.

Reflection Questions

Personal Experience: Which Reproductive Justice tenet have you personally experienced or witnessed in your life? _____

_____

_____

_____

_____

_____

Emotional Response: Which Reproductive Justice tenet makes you feel the most? You might feel excited, hopeless, angry, conflicted, or anything else. _____

_____

_____

_____

_____

_____

Knowledge and Skills: What unique knowledge, skills, or resources do you possess that might be valuable in addressing a specific Reproductive Justice tenet? (For example: Are you a social worker who helps families get care? Or do you work in healthcare, and can change something about your practice?) _____

_____
_____
_____
_____
_____

Community Need: In your specific community, which Reproductive Justice tenet seems most urgent or overlooked? _____

_____
_____
_____
_____
_____

Existing Movements: Are you already involved in other social justice movements? How does your current activism connect to Reproductive Justice? What new connections could you build? _____

_____
_____
_____
_____
_____

Personal Values: Which Reproductive Justice tenet aligns most closely with your core values and beliefs? How does working on this tenet honor what matters most to you?

_____
_____
_____
_____
_____
_____

Impact Assessment: Where do you believe your contribution could make the greatest difference? Consider both the urgency of the need and your capacity to effect change in that area.

_____
_____
_____
_____
_____
_____

Your Turn: Finding Your Place in the Movement

The mission now cannot be to reinstate Roe. Now is the time to embrace a new framework to talk about abortion and access to abortion care. We can't silo abortion care into its own arena, separate from all the other issues impacting people. When we talk about whether or not to bring children into this world, we need to talk about lack of childcare, unsafe housing and neighborhoods, food deserts, unreliable transportation, toxic environments, lack of insurance, and so on.

You can't do it all, but there is a place for everyone:

1. **Direct service providers**: Healthcare providers, doulas, abortion funders, clinic escorts
2. **Community educators**: Sex educators, workshop facilitators, writers, artists
3. **Policy advocates**: Lobbyists, legal advocates, voter mobilization workers
4. **Cultural workers**: Storytellers, religious leaders, media creators
5. **Community organizers**: Coalition builders, grassroots organizers, mutual aid coordinators

Setting Actionable Goals

Based on your skills, experiences, and the pillar of Reproductive Justice that most resonates with you, which role in the movement feels most aligned with your capabilities?

_____
_____
_____
_____
_____
_____
_____
_____

What's one concrete step you can take in the next month to begin fulfilling this role?

_____
_____
_____
_____
_____
_____
_____

Your Commitment to Reproductive Justice

Based on everything you've explored in this chapter, can you articulate your personal commitment to advancing Reproductive Justice?

Your Reproductive Justice Statement:

I am passionate about the Reproductive Justice tenet of _____

because _____

_____

I commit to advancing this tenet by _____

I understand that this work might be challenging because _____

but I am motivated by _____

Chapter 2 Summary

Transformation is a continuous journey. Be patient with yourself through this process. The work of Reproductive Justice requires sustained commitment, community support, and regular reflection.

In the next chapter, we'll explore how to connect the personal to the political, deepening your understanding of how individual experiences shape and are shaped by broader political realities.

Room for Thought

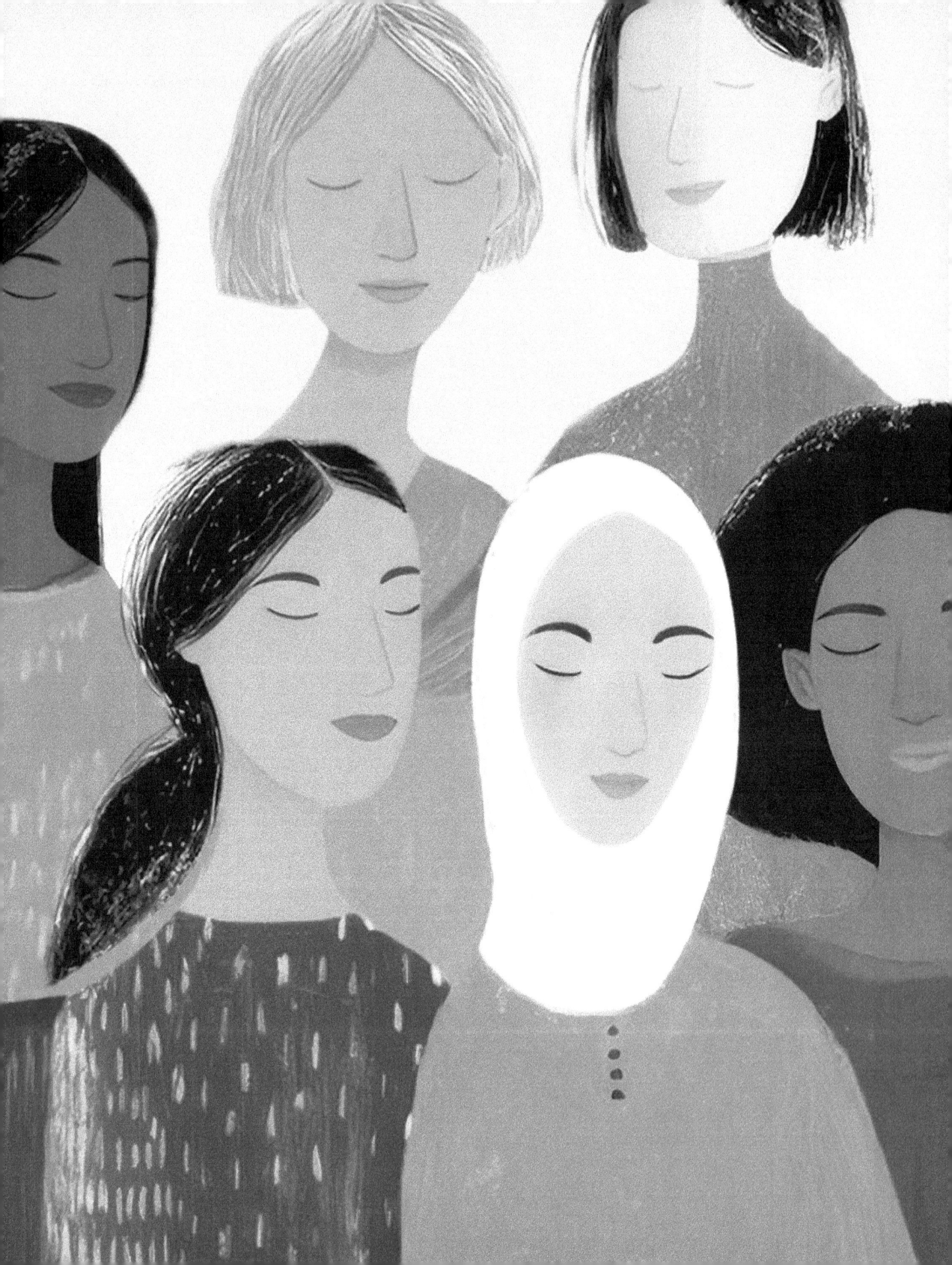

CHAPTER 3

HOW REPRODUCTIVE JUSTICE TOUCHES EVERYTHING

> In what ways does Reproductive Justice intersect with other aspects of your life and community?

Why This Question?

In the previous chapter, we saw why Reproductive Justice isn't just about abortion or contraception, and you identified which tenets of Reproductive Justice spoke to you most.

In this chapter, we'll get more specific by looking at ways Reproductive Justice touches every aspect of our lives. The goal is to show that when we don't silo the abortion debate from other aspects of social, environmental, and economic justice, we find new ways to broaden the Reproductive Justice movement, uniting with advocates for other causes. By the end of this chapter, I hope you'll find the specific intersection of Reproductive Justice and your life that most excites you. So, I ask:

In what ways does Reproductive Justice touch other aspects of your life and community?

Don't worry if you don't see many connections yet. After you've read the chapter, I'll ask you to come back to this list. Hopefully, you'll have uncovered new ways to interact with the movement and advocate with others.

Think about each area below and ask yourself: *"Does this barrier limit a person's ability to decide if, when, or how to build and raise a family?"* The first one is filled in as an example.

Barriers to Deciding If, When, or How to Have and Raise Children

Potential Barrier	Does This Limit Me?	A Loved One?	My Community?
Childcare	**Yes:** I can't afford after-school care, so I'd struggle to work full-time and parent.	**No:** My sister's company offers subsidized on-site daycare, so she always has a spot.	**Yes:** Local daycare centers have long waiting lists and high fees.
Healthcare			
Living Wage			
Paid Family Leave			
Affordable Housing			
Reliable Transportation			
Safe Environment			
Education Access			
Racial Equity			
LGBTQIA Inclusion			
Disability Inclusion			
Political Participation and Voting Rights			

Question for Thought

Looking at the above chart, who is most affected by issues that intersect with Reproductive Justice: you, your loved ones, or your community? Why do you think this is? Does it change the way you think about the intersectional nature of Reproductive Justice?

_____
_____
_____
_____
_____
_____
_____

Our Shared Experience

Those barriers—whether written into law, embedded in economic systems, or enforced by social pressure—are called "reproductive oppression."

Reproductive oppression refers to the regulation and exploitation of a person's body, sexuality, labor, and procreative capacities as a strategy to control individuals and entire communities.

Reproductive oppression isn't accidental. It stems from planned, intentional goals of a culture with a history of slavery, colonization, eugenics, misogyny, and ableism. People's basic rights to decide if, when, and how to have and raise children are blocked by larger forces—laws, policies, social norms, or economic conditions. This is what oppression looks like, and it persists today because we see reproductive issues as separate from housing, policing, environmental justice, or disability rights. Reproductive oppression affects entire communities, especially those already marginalized. When the values and the systems of reproductive oppression go unchallenged, people lose control over their own bodies and their families. Seeing the intersections allows us to better examine our values and how they can unintentionally cause oppression.

Our Shared Values

The stories below illustrate how Reproductive Justice shows up in real life. As you read each scenario, choose which Reproductive Justice pillar is most at stake, then decide whether you think this person is experiencing reproductive oppression. Pay attention to the reasoning behind each answer. It shows different value systems at work.

Rosa's Story

Rosa lost her job when she took unpaid time off for prenatal appointments and was evicted for missing rent, forcing her to choose between shelter and care.

- **Which Reproductive Justice pillar is at stake?**
    - Bodily autonomy
    - The right to have a child
    - The right to not have a child
    - The right to raise a child in a safe environment

- **Is Rosa experiencing reproductive oppression?**
    - **Yes:** People deserve time off for essential healthcare; people deserve safe housing, no matter their income.
    - **No:** Individuals should shoulder personal health needs without social support. Landlords can't support tenants who can't pay.

Michael's Story

Michael lives next to a factory emitting toxic fumes. After his partner's miscarriage, they worry that environmental hazards harmed their ability to carry a pregnancy safely.

- **Which Reproductive Justice pillar is at stake?**
    - Bodily autonomy

- The right to have a child
- The right to not have a child
- The right to raise a child in a safe environment

- **Is Michael experiencing reproductive oppression?**
  - **Yes:** Healthy environments are essential to reproductive freedom.
  - **No:** This is an environmental regulation issue. If they can't afford a safe place to live, they shouldn't have a child; businesses and the jobs they create are more important than passing onerous environmental laws that harm our economy.

Leslie's Story

Leslie and her wife were refused in vitro fertilization (IVF) coverage because their insurer only recognized heterosexual couples as eligible parents.

- **Which Reproductive Justice pillar is at stake?**
  - Bodily autonomy
  - The right to have a child
  - The right to not have a child
  - The right to raise a child in a safe environment

- **Is Leslie experiencing reproductive oppression?**
  - **Yes:** Insurance discrimination blocks her right to have a child on equal terms. Everyone should be seen as equal in the eyes of the law.
  - **No:** Insurers follow existing legal definitions of "family." Why should I have to pay for people who have these sorts of relationships?

Elena's Story

Elena lives 100 miles from the nearest abortion clinic and has no car or public transit option. By the time she found a ride, she'd passed the state's gestational limit and was denied care.

- **Which Reproductive Justice pillar is at stake?**
    - Bodily autonomy
    - The right to have a child
    - The right to not have a child
    - The right to raise a child in a safe environment

- **Is Elena experiencing reproductive oppression?**
    - **Yes:** Lack of transportation stripped her of meaningful choice over her own body and the timing of parenthood. People need support to allow them to access the care they need, and that includes transportation.
    - **No:** This is an infrastructure issue, not a reproductive issue. Reproductive Justice should focus on healthcare.

New Thinking: Social Determinants of Health

When I talk about Reproductive Justice, I'm often talking about the conditions in which people live, work, grow, and age. These conditions have an enormous impact on our health outcomes and are called "social determinants of health." As a doctor providing reproductive healthcare, I see firsthand how these factors can often be more influential than genetics or individual choices on the health outcomes of my patients.

Social determinants of health are the economic and social conditions outside of an individual's control that cause differences in health status.

These factors include:

- Safe housing and neighborhoods
- Access to healthy food

- Transportation reliability
- Clean water and air
- Quality education
- Healthcare access and affordability
- Workplace conditions and job security
- Income and wealth distribution
- Exposure to violence and discrimination

I've seen how these factors dramatically shape my patients' reproductive lives in ways they often don't recognize. The impacts of these social determinants aren't distributed equally. Black people are more susceptible to dying in general and especially in pregnancy and childbirth due to systemic racism and inherent bias. The stress of encountering racism day after day creates what Professor Arline Geronimus calls weathering, "a metaphor that expresses the accumulation of stress from racism in everyday life," which "literally ages Black bodies."[16]

When people say that health is just a personal responsibility, they're missing how these social factors constrain choices. As I've seen in my practice, many people with low incomes can't get to necessary health appointments because of subpar transportation or unreliable childcare. People with low incomes often have employers who are not willing to work with them to provide time off for the frequent appointments that are required for a high-risk pregnancy, so they skip appointments, thus risking their health further.

Environmental factors also significantly impact reproductive health. Exposure to pollution, unsafe drinking water, industrial toxins, and climate change disproportionately affects communities of color and economically disadvantaged neighborhoods. These are the same communities that often have limited access to healthcare.

These social determinants are not accidents but the result of policy choices and systemic inequities. They are why a Reproductive Justice framework is so crucial. It recognizes that the right to have children, not have children, and parent children in safe environments requires addressing these underlying conditions.

Your Social Determinants Profile

Think about the following social determinants of health in your own life and consider how they impact your reproductive autonomy and health. The first one is filled in as an example.

Social Determinant	Me	My Community	How This Impacts My Health & Reproductive Choices	Privilege or Barrier?
Housing stability	I rent an apartment with a fixed one-year lease.	Many neighbors move month-to-month or don't have housing at all.	I can plan prenatal care. People with unstable housing may have difficulty getting to their visits, and because they move from place to place, their provider can lose contact with them.	Privilege
Transportation access				
Food security				
Healthcare access				
Income/Employment				
Environmental quality				
Community safety				
Education				

Which social determinant has the greatest impact on your reproductive health and choices? Why?

How have your social determinants changed throughout your life? How did those changes affect your health options?

Think about someone whose social determinants are very different from yours. How might their reproductive choices and experiences differ from yours as a result?

Who in your community faces the most significant barriers related to social determinants of health? What systems or policies create or maintain these barriers?

_____
_____
_____
_____
_____
_____

What is one social determinant you could help improve—for yourself, someone you care about, or your community? What specific step could you take this month?

_____
_____
_____
_____
_____
_____

My Story

I did a webinar with a couple who needed to travel outside their state to access abortion care for an unviable pregnancy. This is what they told me:

> *It was through the experience of being denied care in our state and then understanding how incredibly lucky we were to be able to surmount the various barriers to getting on a plane last minute, booking last-minute hotels, paying thousands and thousands of dollars out of pocket for the care itself… trying to put all the pieces together in the moment and right away. I mean, we were on that plane thinking, what do people do who don't have a mom to borrow money from?*

Who don't have IDs so they can fly? Who might speak English as a second language?... [We were] going through all of the various privileges that were required for us to surmount this abortion ban that we didn't know existed until we were in the moment and desperately needed care.

A Shift in Thinking: Drawing Connections

How many intersections do the couple in the above story draw between Reproductive Justice and other issues?

- ☐ **Economic privilege**: Having enough money or access to funds for last-minute expenses
- ☐ **Family support systems**: Having family members who can loan money or other aid
- ☐ **Documentation/ID access**: Having a government-issued identification is required for air travel
- ☐ **Language access**: English fluency for navigating medical and travel systems
- ☐ **Transportation access**: Ability to travel across state lines
- ☐ **Time flexibility**: Ability to take time off work, arrange childcare, etc.
- ☐ **Housing security**: After all of the obstacles and barriers faced, there is a home to return to
- ☐ **Geographic location**: Proximity to states with less restrictive laws
- ☐ **Information access**: Knowledge of options and how to navigate complex healthcare systems
- ☐ **Immigration status**: Freedom to travel without fear of detention
- ☐ **Technology access**: Ability to research providers, book travel online
- ☐ **Credit/banking access**: Having credit cards or bank accounts for reservations and payment
- ☐ **Disability status**: Physical ability to endure travel and navigate unfamiliar environments
- ☐ **Healthcare literacy**: Understanding medical terminology and systems

As you review this list, which of these intersections surprised you the most? Which ones might you have overlooked if thinking only about reproductive healthcare in isolation? Which ones affect you? _____

_____
_____
_____
_____
_____

From Thinking to Action: Your Place in the Movement

Reproductive Justice requires all of us. No matter your background, skills, or resources, you have a unique role to play in creating a world where everyone can make reproductive decisions with dignity and support. Because Reproductive Justice touches everything, you can find your place.

Reflection Questions

Personal Experience: After reading this chapter, do you think you've been affected by a social determinant of health, either positively or negatively? _____

_____
_____
_____
_____
_____

Emotional Response: Researchers believe stress can be a social determinant of health. Does that idea resonate with you? Why? _____

_____
_____
_____
_____
_____
_____

Knowledge and Skills: After reading this chapter, what existing knowledge or skills do you possess that could be used to directly address how social determinants of health create systemic barriers in your community? What is one new, actionable skill you feel you need to develop to move from reflection to collective action on this issue? _____

_____
_____
_____
_____
_____
_____

Community Need: In your community, which Reproductive Justice intersection seems most urgent or overlooked? _____

_____
_____
_____
_____
_____
_____

Existing Movements: Does your current activism connect to Reproductive Justice? What new connections could you build?

_____
_____
_____
_____
_____
_____

Personal Values: After reading this chapter, has there been a shift in your thinking between individual and collective values? _____

_____
_____
_____
_____
_____
_____

Impact Assessment: What social determinant of health feels easiest to fix in your community? Hardest? Which would you prefer to tackle? _____

_____
_____
_____
_____
_____
_____

Your Turn

After reflecting on these questions, write a statement identifying which intersection(s) of Reproductive Justice you feel most drawn to and why:

"I feel most connected to the intersection of Reproductive Justice and _____ because _____. My unique contribution to this work could be _____."

If you're still not sure, go back to the original list of intersections between Reproductive Justice and other issues and see if you want to change any answers. If so, which ones and why? Have you thought of any personal stories that arose while reading this chapter that opened your eyes to how Reproductive Justice touches many areas of your life?

Your Personal Commitment to Action

Transformation is incomplete without expression and action. Articulating your new values and goals not only solidifies your understanding but also empowers you to advocate for Reproductive Justice in all its dimensions.

Draft a personal commitment statement summarizing your transformed values and how you plan to live them out. For example:

I am committed to looking beyond single-issue advocacy to address the complex web of factors that affect reproductive autonomy. I am committed to this approach because I believe that until we address these intersecting barriers, reproductive freedom will remain out of reach for many, especially the poorest and most vulnerable people.

Chapter 3 Summary

By understanding Reproductive Justice as connected to all aspects of life—from healthcare access to economic security, from environmental justice to racial equity, from political participation to media literacy—we can build more effective, inclusive movements for change.

Remember that Reproductive Justice requires systemic change, not just individual choices. It demands that we work across movements, building coalitions that address the full spectrum of human needs and rights. It calls us to see Reproductive Justice not as a single issue but as a framework for understanding how power, privilege, and oppression operate in our society.

As you continue your journey, keep asking yourself: How does Reproductive Justice touch everything in my life and community? How can I contribute to creating a world where everyone can make reproductive decisions with dignity, support, and resources? Your voice and your actions matter in this collective struggle for justice.

And now that you see the intersections, we'll look at the most effective way to create change: with political involvement.

Room for Thought

CHAPTER 4

CONNECTING THE PERSONAL TO THE POLITICAL

Do you connect the personal to the political?

Why This Question?

Healthcare, housing, transportation, and other basic needs are shaped by political decisions that can either support or harm you and your community. This connection isn't always obvious. Many of us were taught to view our challenges as purely personal matters that we must solve individually. But recognizing the political dimensions of our experiences opens up new possibilities for collective action and meaningful change.

One way that change happens is on the policy level when harmful government and institutional policies are dismantled and replaced by meaningful systemic change. So, I ask:

Do You Connect the Personal to the Political?

I have seen politics directly affect me when...
_____
_____
_____
_____
_____
_____
_____

I have seen politics directly affect my friends or family when...
_____
_____
_____
_____
_____
_____
_____

Question for Thought

Is it easier to see how politics affects other people's lives than how it affects your own? Why do you think that is or isn't true?
_____
_____
_____
_____
_____

Our Shared Experience

It's hard to connect personal struggles to political systems, and this is by design. When individuals view their challenges as purely personal rather than as the result of deliberate political choices made by their government and institutions, they're less likely to organize for change.

For example, when I ask people to reflect on how politics impacts their daily lives, these are some responses I often hear:

Value Individual Responsibility

- "I can't afford healthcare because insurance is too expensive for me."
- "I can't get time off work to take care of my kids when they're sick."
- "Transportation to medical appointments is difficult to arrange because I don't have a car."
- "I don't have time to travel to the next town to shop for healthier food."

Value Being Part of a Community Controlled by Politics

- "Insurance is expensive because we lack universal healthcare policies."
- "I don't have paid family leave because our lawmakers prioritize business interests over workers."
- "Public transportation is inadequate because of decisions about how tax money is spent."
- "My neighborhood is a food desert because of historical redlining and ongoing disinvestment."

Reflection Exercise

Identify a struggle or a triumph you've had in the past year. _____

_____
_____
_____
_____
_____
_____
_____

How would you talk about this struggle in terms of personal responsibility? _____

_____
_____
_____
_____
_____
_____
_____

How would you rephrase it as influenced by community/policy? _____

_____
_____
_____
_____
_____
_____
_____

Our Shared Values

Often, I hear people say, "I'm not political."

Have you ever said this? If so, what exactly do you mean by it (select all that apply):

☐ I dislike politics. It's too confrontational

☐ I distrust politics. Nothing ever gets done.

☐ I'm not interested in politics. It doesn't affect my life.

☐ I don't have time to keep up with politics. It feels overwhelming.

☐ I feel my vote doesn't matter. Why bother?

☐ I avoid politics so I don't rock the boat with friends or family.

☐ I find political debates divisive and stressful.

☐ I think all politicians are corrupt or self-serving.

☐ I believe politics is only for experts or insiders.

☐ I feel powerless to influence any political outcome.

☐ I'd rather focus on direct action in my community than on distant governments.

Which of the reasons for not being political most resonates with you? How does that influence your willingness or unwillingness to get involved in politics?

_____
_____
_____
_____
_____
_____
_____

New Thinking: Your Health Is Political

In the previous chapter, you saw that social determinants of health are the economic and social conditions outside of an individual's control that cause differences in health status. Racism, poverty, unsafe neighborhoods, unhealthy food, toxic environments, and so on are all social determinants of health that contribute to obesity, diabetes, high blood pressure, and other conditions that make pregnancy and childbirth more dangerous.

These social determinants aren't accidents—they're the result of political policies. By engaging in politics, we can structurally change these areas of our lives.

Access to Healthcare

In April 2020, researchers found that in periods during and after pregnancy, all categories of minority women experienced higher rates of uninsurance than White, non-Latine women.

The disparity was significant:

- 75.3 percent of White, non-Latine women were continually insured
- 55.4 percent of Black, non-Latine women were continually insured
- 49.9 percent of Indigenous women were continually insured
- 20.5 percent of Latine, Spanish-speaking women were continually insured[17]

I've seen clearly in my practice that being uninsured contributes to worse health outcomes for pregnant people and their infants. People miss appointments, discontinue care, or never show up at all.

What feelings come up when you consider pregnant individuals and their infants going without health insurance?

Based on the data showing who is most often uninsured, what specific goal should a new insurance policy prioritize to reduce the disparity for Black, Indigenous, and Latine women?

Thinking about your answer to the previous question, what government office or legislative body (e.g., state legislature, Congress, the Governor's Office) has the authority to make that goal a reality?

Does this issue interest you enough to get involved in the politics of health insurance? Which of these actions would you consider:

- Contact your representatives to urge them to expand Medicaid, remove eligibility caps, or create a public option—a government-provided health insurance plan that competes with private health insurance companies.
- Sign or start a petition calling for state or federal reforms to guarantee continuous prenatal and postpartum coverage.
- Speak up at town halls or city council meetings about the harms of uninsured pregnancy.

Localizing Reproductive Justice

The overturning of *Roe v. Wade* demonstrates how political decisions directly affect our most intimate choices. Supreme Court Justice Samuel Alito, the lead writer of the Dobbs decision that overturned Roe, told us that the power now lies with the states and each of their individual electorates. Now, we have to go out state-by-state, ballot-measure-by-ballot-measure, election-by-election, and take control of that power.

What emotions arise for you when you think about state-level bans on abortion care?

_____
_____
_____
_____
_____
_____

Beyond voting, what are some strategies or public campaigns that grassroots activists and organizations could use to fight restrictive abortion laws at the state or local level?

_____
_____
_____
_____
_____
_____

When it comes to reproductive rights, which officials at the state level and the local level hold the most power to either prevent new bans or lessen the impact of existing restrictive laws?

_____
_____
_____
_____
_____
_____

Does this issue interest you enough to get involved in the politics of abortion bans? Which of these actions would you consider?

- Attend candidate forums and ask where they stand on abortion policy.
- Vote for candidates who pledge to defend abortion rights.
- Testify at state legislative hearings to oppose restrictive abortion bills.
- Research whether your state has a ballot initiative campaign to enshrine the right to abortion care in your state constitution.

Pregnancy Criminalization

When strict abortion laws are passed, normal biological events such as miscarriage become criminalized. Miscarriage is not unusual:

- 15 to 20 percent of pregnancies end in miscarriage; pregnancy loss before the twentieth week[18]
- One in 160 births ends in stillbirth; pregnancy loss after the twentieth week—24,000 babies a year.[19]
- Another 4 in 1,000 infants die in the first twenty-eight days of life, usually due to premature birth, low birthweight, and birth defects.[20]

As anti-abortion laws increase, every one of these losses becomes a potential criminal event. The National Advocates for Pregnant Women reports that pregnancy criminalization has more than tripled from 2006 through 2020.[21]

In addition, the Centers for Disease Control and Prevention (CDC) reports that stillbirths are more common in Black pregnant people and those from low socioeconomic communities. Non-Latine Black people have 2.3 times the infant mortality rate as non-Latine Whites.[22]

What emotions arise for you when you think about pregnancy criminalization? _____

_____
_____
_____
_____
_____

Thinking about your community, what are the two most urgent changes you believe would protect people from being criminalized after a miscarriage or stillbirth?

_____
_____
_____
_____
_____
_____

Who are the key decision-makers who could stop or reverse the criminalization of pregnancy at the local level (like a District Attorney or City Council) and the state level (like the Governor or Attorney General)?

_____
_____
_____
_____
_____

Does this issue interest you enough to get involved in the politics of pregnancy criminalization? Which of these actions might you consider:

- Support bail funds and legal defense for those criminalized for their pregnancy outcomes
- Advocate for legislation that explicitly protects people from prosecution for pregnancy outcomes
- Educate healthcare providers about their role in preventing pregnancy criminalization

Comprehensive Sex Education

There is no federal requirement that sex ed be taught in schools, so, as with abortion rights, we face a patchwork of rules and requirements. Beyond some general state guidelines, decisions about sexual education are made by individual school districts. The consequences of inadequate sex education are significant:

- In the United States, 20 percent of thirteen- to fourteen-year-olds and 44 percent of fifteen- to seventeen-year-olds reported that they had "some type of romantic relationship or dating experience."[23]
- Many states, including Arizona, where I live and practice, provide state funding for abstinence-only education, which doesn't work.
- Many states pass laws to prohibit school districts from providing comprehensive sex education to their students or jeopardize their funding.

What feelings come up when you think of the sex education you were taught in school? How about your children? Were there things you wished were or weren't addressed?

_____
_____
_____
_____
_____
_____
_____
_____
_____
_____
_____
_____

What is the single biggest policy or funding barrier standing in the way of better sex education where you live, and what is one action you could take to address it?

_____
_____
_____
_____
_____
_____

To get the kind of comprehensive sex education you want, who currently has the authority to approve, block, or fund the school curriculum in your district and state? *(Consider: Who signs the bill into law? Who votes on the budget?)*

_____
_____
_____
_____
_____
_____

Does this issue interest you enough to get involved in the politics of sex education? Which of these activities might you consider:

- Connect with parent groups advocating for evidence-based sex education
- Attend school board meetings when sex education curriculum is discussed
- Support organizations that provide sex education outside school settings
- Run to be a local school board member

Climate Safety and Environmental Justice

People cannot raise families in safe, sustainable communities when those communities are threatened by pollution, extreme weather, and resource depletion. Environmental conditions are social determinants of health that directly influence reproductive outcomes.

Not surprisingly, climate change and environmental injustice disproportionately impact those with the fewest resources to adapt, often people marginalized by race, class, and geography.

The connections between climate justice and Reproductive Justice include:

- **Environmental toxins and reproductive health**: Pollution and environmental contaminants contribute to infertility, pregnancy complications, and poor maternal and infant health outcomes.
- **Climate displacement**: As climate change makes regions uninhabitable, families are forced to relocate, disrupting healthcare access and community support networks.
- **Resource access**: Climate change threatens access to clean water, nutritious food, and safe shelter—all essential for reproductive health and family well-being.
- **Intergenerational justice**: Decisions about whether to have children include considerations about what kind of world those children will inherit.

What feelings come up when you think of the environmental conditions of your community? Are there areas that need urgent action? _____

_____
_____
_____
_____
_____
_____
_____
_____

To address the most urgent environmental issues in your community, what kind of reform or regulation do you think is needed most? _____

_____

_____

_____

_____

_____

_____

Thinking about that needed reform, where does the power to make it happen primarily lie (e.g., The Mayor's Office, a state legislative committee, the EPA, a local community council, etc.)? _____

_____

_____

_____

_____

_____

_____

Does this issue interest you enough to get involved in the politics of climate change? Which of these actions might you consider:

- Join environmental justice organizations in your community
- Advocate for clean air and water protection in vulnerable neighborhoods
- Support the development of climate resilience plans that center reproductive health
- Connect climate activism to Reproductive Justice in public discussions

Family Leave and Support Policies

Political decisions determine what kind of support families receive, creating very different experiences based on who you are. Federal law mandates only twelve weeks of unpaid family leave for pregnancy, birth, and childcare combined. Most people with low incomes can't afford to take advantage of this unpaid leave, and strict eligibility requirements make it so that less than two-thirds of the US workforce is even eligible. The people with service jobs who have to interact with customers all day, or people with jobs on their feet like waitresses, nurses, or retail workers, are often the least likely to be able to use their leave, and also the people most likely to find it impossible to fight back mild nausea or other symptoms while also doing their jobs.

What feelings come up when you think of the support available to families raising children? Have you taken advantage of these supports or been denied them? _____
_____
_____
_____
_____
_____
_____

What changes to laws or policies do you think would make the biggest difference in the lives of families raising children?_____
_____
_____
_____
_____
_____
_____

Which public officials at the federal and state levels would need to act to create these reforms?

_____
_____
_____
_____
_____
_____
_____

Does this issue interest you enough to get involved in the politics of paid family and caregiver leave? Which of the following actions might you consider:

- Reach out to your federal and state representatives to urge the passage of paid family leave legislation.
- Offer to testify at state legislative hearings in support of expanding family leave benefits, lending a personal voice to the issue.
- Urge your governor to use their authority to issue an executive order that expands leave eligibility for state employees or contractors.
- Research and vote for candidates at every level who make paid family and caregiver leave a top priority in their campaigns.

My Story

When I arrived in Phoenix in 2009, Arizona was in the process of unleashing a wave of sweeping anti-abortion bills. As the years passed, the pattern soon felt ritualistic: every year, there was one more restriction, one more barrier constricting access, making it nearly impossible for people to get timely essential care.

What was going on here?

To find out, I got involved in the political process at the local level, and I learned that policy was being written in a vacuum, sealed off from lived experience. Not a single person deciding the fate of abortion care had ever had or provided one, had more than a passing knowledge of medicine, or was even still within their reproductive years. Nor did any of them stand where my patients stood: marginalized due to race, religion, socioeconomic status, and other factors.

In other words, no laws enacted by the legislature had much of an effect on their own lives.

During my first year trying to influence politics, I saw thirteen anti-abortion bills introduced and twelve defeated. While that might sound great, the bill that slipped through would cause real harm, especially piled onto the bill that had slipped through the year before, and the year before, and so on.

This was how change happened: slowly, deliberately, and under the radar.

Until that moment, I had been content as an advocate—someone who speaks out about harm to others. My white coat had earned me a hearing, but watching thirteen attacks distilled to one crucial loss showed me the limits of distance. We needed more voices in the direct, political fight. If lawmakers wouldn't invite patients and providers into the conversation, we had to shoulder our way in. Speaking about the people affected was no longer enough; I needed to stand with them.

Over the next years, I transformed from an advocate to a political activist. I vowed to find a way in which those who live with the consequences of reproductive policy were the ones shaping it.

My personal evolution from being a physician who was an ally for my patients to becoming a political activist for my community was inspired by my deep involvement with the community. My interest in Reproductive Justice grew as I served and worked with organizations that were working to better the conditions of that community. Once I saw the impact that politics could have on the conditions of my patients' lives, I knew that my mission was so much bigger than doing a pelvic exam or Pap smear. I saw all the ways in which I could make a real difference.

DID YOU KNOW?

Allies support the movement through private conversations, donations, letters to lawmakers, social media posts, or petitions.

Advocates speak publicly, educate others, attend rallies, fundraise, and join organizations.

Activists organize and mobilize communities, maintain sustained engagement, and often put themselves on the line alongside directly impacted people.

These roles aren't fixed, and the movement needs people at all levels. What matters is engaging where you are, with your current skills and capacity.

A Shift in Thinking: From Individual to Political Values

Understanding the connection between the personal and political requires shifting our perspective on values that many of us have internalized. Here are some transformative shifts in thinking:

Original (Individual) Values	Emerging (Collective) Values
Personal responsibility for all outcomes	Recognition of systemic barriers and shared responsibility
Politics is separate from daily life	Politics shapes our everyday experiences
Voting is the only political action	Multiple ways to engage politically (organizing, educating, etc.)
My voice doesn't matter	Collective voices create change
If it doesn't affect me directly, it's not my concern	Solidarity with others whose struggles are different but connected
Change happens only at the individual level	Systems can and must be transformed
Political discussions are impolite or divisive	Political engagement is necessary for community well-being
Healthcare is a consumer product	Healthcare is a human right
My reproductive choices are private	Reproductive freedom requires public support

When we see issues through this collective lens, we acknowledge that some people don't have a choice because they and their communities are being oppressed.

Question for Thought

Do your values fall more to the left or the right of the chart? _____

_____
_____
_____
_____
_____
_____

From Thinking to Action: Finding Your Voice

Now that you see the connections between your personal experiences and political systems, how can you use this understanding to create change? Here are some ways to engage:

At the Personal Level

- Educate yourself about the political dimensions of the issues you care about
- Share your story and listen to others' experiences
- Vote in every election, especially local ones that directly impact your community

The state legislature is where laws are made, whether about abortion, voter suppression, or other issues that matter. We have to continue to fight to be in a position where we have the power.

Within Your Community

- Join local organizations working on issues you care about
- Attend town halls and community meetings
- Support candidates who prioritize your community's needs
- Have conversations with family and friends about these connections

Everyone must find their own way to show up, considering their specific conditions, skills, and talents. There are so many ways to get involved and support the cause of advancing reproductive health, rights, and justice. There's a place for everyone at this moment. There are many different ways to fight back.

At the Systemic Level

- Contact your representatives about specific policies
- Organize with others for collective action
- Support litigation and policy advocacy efforts
- Use your professional expertise to advocate for better systems

Reflection Questions

Personal Experience: Now that you've read this chapter, have you seen more ways that the personal is political in your life? _____

_____

_____

_____

_____

_____

Emotional Response: How did the information in this chapter make you feel? More vulnerable or more powerful? Why?

_____
_____
_____
_____
_____
_____

Knowledge and Skills: Do you have any specific skills that might make you a valuable political activist? For example, are you a healthcare practitioner, or has your experience given you a story to tell?

_____
_____
_____
_____
_____
_____

Community Need: In your community, what is the most urgent issue that policy change could solve?

_____
_____
_____
_____
_____
_____

Existing Movements: Do you know of or are you already involved in other politically active groups? For example, are you part of a church group or women's group where your stories could be useful, or could you harness these groups to focus on this issue?

_____
_____
_____
_____
_____
_____
_____

Personal Values: Which values have been most challenged by the ideas in this chapter? How does that make you feel? _____

_____
_____
_____
_____
_____
_____
_____

Impact Assessment: Where do you believe your contribution could make the greatest difference in changing policy? Consider both the need and your capacity to effect change in that area. _____

_____
_____
_____
_____
_____
_____

Your Turn

Draft a Personal Action Plan

Based on what you've learned, create an action plan for connecting your personal experiences to political change:

My sphere of influence: (Check all that apply)

- ☐ Family/friends
- ☐ Workplace/professional network
- ☐ Neighborhood/local community
- ☐ Faith community
- ☐ Online networks
- ☐ Other: _____

Actions I will take in the next month: _____

1. _____

2. _____

3. _____

Resources I need: _____

Potential allies: _____

_____
_____
_____
_____
_____

The Power of Your Story

Your personal experiences are powerful tools for political change. When we share our stories with others, we help them see the connections between individual struggles and systemic issues. When I speak with politicians, they do appreciate hearing from me as a clinician, but hearing stories directly from impacted people in the community carries more weight.

Your stories matter. Telling them to the right people can make a huge difference in creating a world in which more people have reproductive equity in their lives.

Exercise: Crafting Your Story

Think about a personal experience you've had that connects to a broader political issue: access to healthcare, abortion, pregnancy criminalization, sex education, climate and environmental justice, family leave and support, or any other issue. Use these prompts to develop a compelling narrative:

What happened? (Briefly describe the experience) _____

_____
_____
_____
_____
_____

How did it affect you personally?

What systems or policies contributed to this situation?

What change would have made a difference?

How could sharing this story help politicians better understand the issue?

_____
_____
_____
_____
_____
_____

Chapter 4 Summary

We're in a moment when simply being angry is no longer enough. It is imperative that each of us define a vision and then find a path. Choose your own level of comfort and identify the options and issues that are in your wheelhouse. Then, stretch yourself a bit. The magic truly happens when you push past your comfort zone. There is something you can do right now based on your life situation, skills, intelligence, financial means, location, and more. Each of us must reflect on the social problems we face, informed by our personal experiences, and commit to learning more about them, sharing what we discover, and finding ways to get involved to push for change. The time for passive hope is over. Someone else will not do it. The courts will not handle it. We are the ones who will save us.

In the next chapters, we'll explore how faith and culture shape our understanding of Reproductive Justice, and how to navigate difficult conversations with those who may not share our values.

Room for Thought

CASE STUDY

THE CRIMINALIZATION OF PREGNANCY LOSS: THE BRITTANY WATTS STORY

> "I don't want any other woman to go through what I had to go through."
> —Brittany Watts[24]

Brittany Watts, a Black, thirty-four-year-old medical receptionist from Warren, Ohio, was twenty-one weeks and five days pregnant when her water broke. The fetus's lungs were far too immature to sustain life outside the womb. Fetal lung maturity is typically sufficient to support a premature birth around thirty-two weeks, and most hospitals will not initiate intensive care before twenty-three weeks. In other words, when her water broke, Brittany's fetus had become non-viable. Meaning it could not live inside the uterus without fluid and could not survive outside the womb.

The accepted treatment in a case like this is to induce labor or perform a dilation and evacuation procedure to end the pregnancy safely before infection, sepsis, or hemorrhage can develop, potentially fatal complications once the pregnant person's water or amniotic sac has broken. Once the water has broken, the barrier to the uterus is gone, making the pregnant person highly susceptible to sepsis. Waiting for a fever or other signs of advanced infection before intervening is often too late and medically negligent, which is why immediate delivery is typically required. The anticipated and tragic outcome when delivery is induced for a non-viable fetus is a stillbirth or fetal demise, depending on the specific gestational age and legal requirements. The fetus is typically delivered without signs of life or survives only a few minutes. This treatment focuses on the pregnant person's survival while acknowledging the inevitable loss of the fetus. In states with abortion bans and restrictions, doctors' medical ethics are often at odds with the legal ramifications of providing necessary care.

Although doctors reported that Brittany's white blood cell count had more than doubled and warned she needed immediate treatment to avoid being "on death's door," Mercy Health St. Joseph Hospital did not induce labor. In Ohio, there are criminal penalties for any procedure that "purposely terminates" a pregnancy after twenty-one weeks and six days if the fetus still has a heartbeat. Thus, doctors worried that induction could be deemed an abortion because a fetus with a heartbeat would be expelled.

According to Brittany, they left her waiting without care or information for hours while the hospital's "ethics" committee deliberated. A report was finally issued giving consent for induction, but hours later, care still wasn't given. Eventually, alone, frightened, untreated, and in pain, Brittany went home against the doctor's orders. According to Brittany, the medical staff at the hospital never told her why it was taking so long to get care.

Two days later, Brittany miscarried alone in her bathroom. Still bleeding hours later, she returned to the hospital. A nurse consoled her, then called the police. Officers went to Brittany's home, unbolted her toilet from the bathroom floor, and carried it away so the medical examiner could retrieve the fetus's remains, which were caught in the trap.

A few weeks later, on October 5, police officers came to Brittany's home, put her in handcuffs, and arrested her for abuse of a corpse, a fifth-degree felony that carries up to a year in jail.

For the next three months, she juggled court hearings, postpartum recovery, fear for her future, extensive legal fees, and grief over her pregnancy loss. In January 2024, a Trumbull County grand jury refused to indict her, and she was never prosecuted on criminal charges.

Watts is now suing the hospital, its parent company, Bon Secours Mercy Health, the city of Warren, and individual police officers and nurses involved, claiming violations of her constitutional rights, medical negligence, violation of privacy laws, and emotional distress. All parties have denied wrongdoing. According to Watts's GoFundMe page, she is devoting herself to full-time advocacy work, claiming her "power, passion, and possibilities."

What thoughts or feelings did Brittany's story bring up for you?

Take a moment to write down your immediate emotional response to this story.

_____
_____
_____
_____
_____
_____
_____
_____

Do you think the doctors in this story made the right call? Why or why not?

_____
_____
_____
_____
_____
_____

How do you view the nurse's decision to contact the police?

And the police? What are your thoughts about their actions?

Imagine your loved one in Brittany's situation. What might you have done if you had been in the emergency room with her, waiting for care?

Stories of Reproductive Oppression

Sometime in April 2024, I was at the Pride Rainbows Festival in Phoenix. A Black woman hesitantly walked by the table. I wasn't sure she was going to stop, but then she did. It took her a while to speak, and she didn't make eye contact at first. But eventually she said, "I used to be pro-life, but I don't think people should be criminalized for their miscarriages." Then she looked up and said, "I don't know if I'm pro…" She choked on the word "choice," unable to get it out. Still, I was heartened by the interaction. She had been staunchly pro-life, but now, seeing what's happening, she was moved to re-evaluate her stance.

Stories move people. The criminalization of miscarriage especially moves people.

This is a phenomenon that I see often. People think that laws are fair and reasonable because they never think much about them. Laws are cold and abstract. But hearing real, emotional stories of grieving people put in handcuffs while the police rip out their plumbing—*Can you imagine?*—pushes them to recognize that increasing criminalization of pregnancy has terrible consequences. It makes them understand, *This could happen to me or someone I love.*

To create a better world, we need to envision it, take action, and convince others to join us. The first and last step—envisioning and persuading—is done most powerfully through listening and storytelling. We can share, with consent, the stories of our friends, family, loved ones, community members, and even strangers like Brittany. These stories are important tools to change people's minds and create the world we want to live in. As sad, maddening, and challenging as Brittany's story is, it can point us to a vision of what could have gone right and how things could be better.

Stories inspire hope and drive action. They help us imagine different outcomes (envision), retell the story to others (unify), and work toward a world where those better outcomes can become reality (action). For example, envision a world in which:

The doctors could have...

What would need to change for this to become a reality?

The nurses could have...

What would need to change for this to become a reality?
_____
_____
_____
_____
_____
_____
_____
_____

The police could have…
_____
_____
_____
_____
_____
_____
_____
_____

What would need to change for this to become a reality?
_____
_____
_____
_____
_____
_____
_____
_____

The legal system could have...

What would need to change for this to become a reality?

Reflection: Do you think that there is anything that Brittany could have done to change the outcome of her situation?

The Intersections of Reproductive Oppression

Brittany's story is a story of the intersectional nature of reproductive oppression.

A quick reminder: **Reproductive oppression is a means of selectively controlling the destiny of entire communities through the bodies of women and individuals. This control operates through interconnected systems that work together to limit reproductive freedom and autonomy.**

Some of the systems of oppression intersecting in Brittany's story are:

Healthcare System

- An ethics committee delaying life-saving care
- Doctors prioritizing potential legal consequences over patient needs
- Nobody explaining to Brittany why her care was delayed

Criminal Justice System

- Police treating a pregnancy loss as a potential crime
- Forcibly removing private property (her toilet) during a medical crisis
- Handcuffing and arresting a woman who had just experienced pregnancy loss

Economic System

- Four months of disruption to Brittany's life and livelihood
- Legal fees requiring a GoFundMe campaign
- Potential long-term employment consequences of an arrest record

State Surveillance System

- Turning medical providers into extensions of law enforcement
- Treating pregnancy outcomes as matters for police intervention
- Creating fear that prevents people from seeking necessary care

Media and Public Narrative

- Trauma of experiencing public legal persecution while grieving
- Public shame and judgment during a deeply personal crisis

Reflection Questions

Which of these systems of oppression surprised you most in Brittany's story? Remember, systems are made up of people, so this question is really asking whose behavior surprised you most? _____

_____

_____

_____

_____

_____

_____

Do you see these different systems reinforcing and amplifying each other? For example, do you think the medical community and law enforcement community were in partnership or opposition? _____

_____

_____

_____

_____

_____

Which systems do you think are most important to address first, and why?

_____
_____
_____
_____
_____
_____
_____

My Reflections

Doctors like me and other healthcare providers are being co-opted into participating in state actions targeting pregnant people. I believe that healthcare workers should not cooperate with law enforcement.

As the main institutional contact with pregnant people, my job as a medical and medical-adjacent provider is to welcome, protect, and help people, not to surveil and potentially criminalize them. I am not an extension of the state. When I became a doctor, I took an oath to do no harm. When I allow myself to be co-opted into the police and carceral state, I am acting against that oath.

Members of the healthcare community can fight against increased criminalization of healthcare by following the "do no harm" principles set out by decriminalization advocates.[25] From the important work of these advocates, I've identified four main principles for my personal day-to-day clinical work and my personal activism:

1. Don't call law enforcement on suspicion of "illegal" behavior.

Our job is to provide healthcare. Contacting law enforcement when we suspect people of having ended pregnancies "illegally" becomes another reason for people who need care to avoid seeking it, leading to worse outcomes. Bringing law enforcement into the healthcare environment is almost never the right choice.

2. Fight against the US Immigration and Customs Enforcement (ICE) presence in hospitals and in or near healthcare facilities.

ICE officials have no place in healthcare environments. We know that even lawful immigrants are increasingly fearful of interactions with police and ICE, and thus, when they worry about these forces' presence, they avoid seeking care.[26] In order to protect patients from ICE presence, providers should be aware of their rights. This area of law is constantly changing and can be regional, but in general, healthcare clinics are considered "sensitive locations" where ICE activity is limited. Providers should be wary of collecting immigration status information and be aware of what documents are in public view in case of ICE presence.

3. Don't support prosecution in cases against people who manage their own care.

The majority of people who manage their own abortion care do so successfully. Medication abortion is extremely safe and effective, and many people are able to perform it with little to no professional intervention. Other ways to self-induce abortions can be less safe and effective, but people still turn to these methods in situations of desperation when no other care is available. When something does go wrong, people need to feel safe to go to emergency rooms or other providers for help. When we criminalize these people, they won't access care, causing unnecessary injury, illness, or even death. Committing to providing care with no questions asked is crucial in keeping people safe.

4. Organize against substandard care in jails, prisons, and detention facilities.

Pregnant people deserve to serve their time and get the care they need in dignity. Women are the fastest-growing population in American prisons, and 80 percent of women in jail are already mothers.[27] Thus, we need to really think as healthcare providers about what it means when women and mothers go to jail. The ultimate solution is to stop trying to solve social problems with incarceration, and that should be a focus of activism. Until that day, we, as medical providers, need to lend our voices to support advocates.

By adopting these principles and sharing our stories, I believe we can dismantle the oppressive narratives that trap people within unjust systems.

Have you ever experienced a situation in which a physician did or didn't uphold these standards? What happened, and how did it make you feel? _____

_____
_____
_____
_____
_____
_____
_____

Your Turn

Do you have a story about reproductive oppression that might change people's minds—either your own, a loved one's, a community member's, or something you saw in the news?

While tragic cases like Brittany's are absolutely heartbreaking and deserve attention, we must also ensure we don't overshadow the equally powerful everyday stories of reproductive oppression that often go untold. These stories may not garner online clicks, yet they are crucial for changing hearts and minds. They also frequently serve as the underlying context within a major news story like Brittany's.

For example:

- Was there a time medical professionals didn't tell you what was going on with your care?
- Was there a time you left a healthcare setting without care because you felt ignored or forgotten?
- Have you had a miscarriage and weren't given adequate emotional support?
- Were you ever afraid of the authorities in a healthcare situation?

These everyday experiences may seem less dramatic than handcuffs and criminal charges, but they represent the same systems of oppression at work. When we share these stories, we help others see the connections between high-profile cases like Brittany's and the more common experiences that shape reproductive health outcomes every day.

What story can you share?

Who might you tell this story to? How would they benefit?

Which systems intersect in your story (healthcare, economic, legal, etc.)? How do they reinforce each other?

What would Reproductive Justice look like in your story? What changes to policy, practice, or community support would have made a difference?

_____
_____
_____
_____
_____
_____
_____
_____
_____
_____
_____

From Vision to Unity to Action

Storytelling is just the start. Here are a few actions you can take when addressing the intersections of criminalizing pregnancy and other systems, including resources for getting started. Which feels right to you?

- Engage in open and honest conversations with loved ones, colleagues, and community members.
- Advocate for policies that expand access to reproductive healthcare. (In Our Own Voice provides an annual policy agenda: https://blackrj.org/wp-content/uploads/2025/06/2025-Black-Reproductive-Justice-Policy-Agenda_In-Our-Own-Voice-2025.pdf.)
- Learn more about how racial bias in healthcare settings leads to pregnancy criminalization in communities already marginalized. (Pregnancy Justice at https://www.pregnancyjusticeus.org)

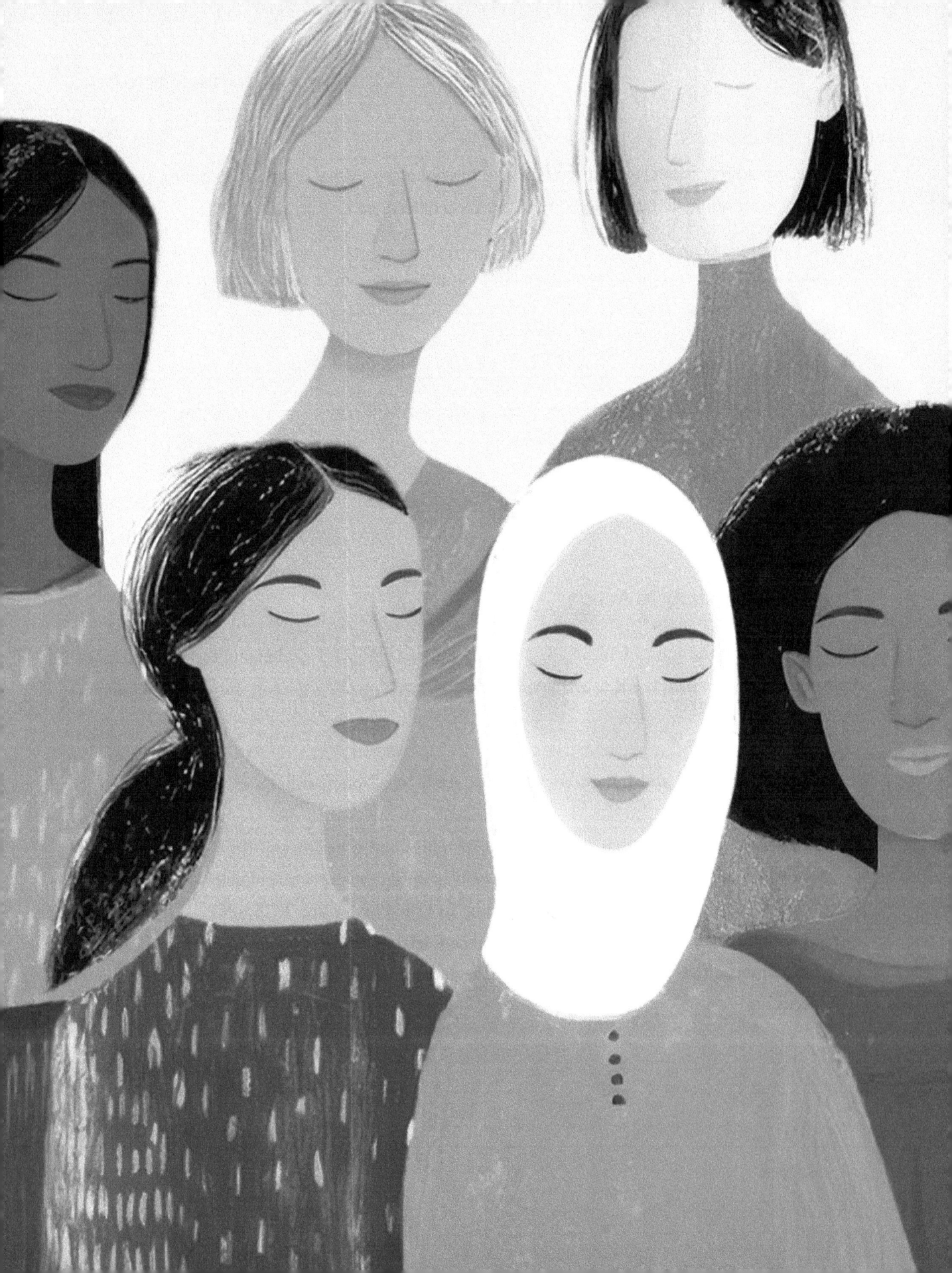

CHAPTER 5

FAITH AND ABORTION CARE

Is there a place for faith in abortion care?

Why This Question?

I get more reactions—both positive and negative—when I discuss faith and abortion care than any other issue. Opening the door to honest and compassionate dialogue about the complex ways in which faith and reproductive health intersect invites us to confront the stigma, silence, and judgment that can sometimes surround abortion within faith communities, as well as the joy and inclusion that Reproductive Justice can bring to the issue. Faith often becomes a proxy for political power grabs in ways that can be hard to untangle. So, I ask:

Is there a place for faith in abortion care?

In your faith tradition, what have you been taught about abortion?

Have other groups' spiritual beliefs shaped your views on abortion?

Question for Thought

If your faith tradition teaches that abortion is wrong, do you believe there are circumstances in which it might be acceptable for you? What about for someone who does not practice the same faith as you?

Our Shared Experience

Each of us brings something different to the intersection of faith and abortion. For some, faith is a source of comfort, clarity, or guidance. For others, it may be a source of tension, confusion, or silence. Even within the same faith tradition, there can be a wide range of interpretations and beliefs. Exploring these differences with openness and respect allows us to move beyond assumptions and toward greater understanding and compassion for ourselves and for others.

Reflection Exercise

Consider the following statements and mark whether you **Agree**, **Disagree**, or are **Unsure**.

Reflection statement	Agree	Disagree	Unsure
My faith tradition has a clearly defined position on abortion.			
My religious beliefs play a significant role in how I view abortion.			
Even though I hold strong personal beliefs about abortion, I don't think those beliefs should be imposed on others.			
I believe that life begins at conception.			
I have encountered different opinions within my faith community regarding abortion.			
I believe a person's religious beliefs should guide their decision-making around abortion.			
I think religious leaders have a responsibility to provide guidance on abortion.			
I feel that my faith community provides a safe space for open, nonjudgmental dialogue about abortion.			
I am open to understanding how people of differing faiths, or none, view abortion.			
Most people who oppose abortion are religious and speak for most people of faith.			
It is possible to hold religious values and support access to abortion care.			
People of faith typically don't get abortion care.			

Our Shared Values

Our underlying cultural values about abortion are often shaped by deeper, often unspoken values that come from our families, our faith communities, and the broader culture around us. These values can be so deeply embedded, we're often not aware of their existence. Sometimes, these values can offer a sense of moral clarity, but they can also create pressure, shame, or confusion, especially when someone is facing a difficult reproductive health decision.

Examples of Underlying Values

Motherhood as a Central Role

In many faith communities, motherhood is deeply honored and seen as a sacred calling. This value can shape the belief that bearing and raising children is a woman's highest purpose, and that choosing not to become a parent—or to end a pregnancy—runs counter to that role.

Do you hold this value? How has it influenced your views or expectations around parenting and reproductive decisions?

_____
_____
_____
_____
_____
_____
_____
_____
_____
_____
_____
_____
_____

Sexual Activity and Moral Behavior

Some traditions teach that sexual activity should only occur within marriage and that an unplanned pregnancy outside of that context reflects a lapse in moral behavior. This belief may influence how abortion is viewed—not only as a medical decision, but also as a response to perceived wrongdoing.

Have you encountered this value in your community or upbringing? How does it shape your understanding of unplanned pregnancy and abortion?

_____
_____
_____
_____
_____

Sacrifice and Spiritual Growth

Certain faith traditions emphasize the spiritual importance of enduring hardship for the sake of others. In this light, carrying a pregnancy to term, regardless of personal cost, may be seen as a meaningful sacrifice. This value can offer strength and purpose, but may also feel limiting or overwhelming in some situations.

Is this a value you relate to? How do you balance ideas of sacrifice with care for your own well-being or that of your family?

_____
_____
_____
_____
_____

The Value of Conception

Some people believe that life begins at conception and that this belief calls for the protection of what has been termed "the unborn." This value can guide deeply held convictions and influence both personal decisions and broader views on abortion.

Do you believe that life begins at conception? If so, do you believe there's any opportunity to reconcile this belief with the complex realities individuals face when making reproductive decisions? _____

_____

_____

_____

_____

_____

_____

_____

New Thinking: How Reproductive Justice Aligns with Religious Values

At first glance, faith and abortion might seem to be in conflict if we are influenced by the dominant social narratives around abortion. However, when we view the issue through the lens of Reproductive Justice, we discover powerful alignment between the values that guide many faith traditions—compassion, dignity, and justice—and the principles that underpin this movement.

In other words, the tenets of Reproductive Justice are not only political. They are moral, ethical, and for many, deeply spiritual.

1. The Right to Bodily Autonomy

Bodily autonomy is the right to make decisions about your own body, free from violence, shame, or coercion. Many faith traditions, including Christianity, teach that people are created in the image of God and are called to seek wisdom through prayer, reflection, and conscience. Reproductive Justice honors that sacred responsibility—the belief that individuals can listen to God in their hearts and decide what is right for them.

2. The Right to Have Children

Reproductive oppression has long denied certain communities, especially Black, Indigenous, disabled, immigrant, and people with low incomes, the freedom to have and raise children. From forced sterilizations to family separation, these injustices persist today. Reproductive Justice affirms the right to parent with dignity and support. Many faith traditions uphold the sanctity of family and call for justice, care, and community. When faith communities defend this right, they live out those values in powerful ways.

3. The Right Not to Have Children

Sometimes, choosing *not* to have a child is an act of love, wisdom, or protection. Reproductive Justice supports the right to make that decision without shame. Faith traditions that honor compassion, discernment, and personal responsibility can—and often do—affirm that people of faith are capable of making thoughtful, moral decisions about whether and when to become parents.

4. The Right to Raise Children in Safe and Sustainable Communities

Raising a child requires more than love—it requires safe neighborhoods, clean water, stable housing, and communities free from violence and discrimination. Reproductive Justice calls out the systemic barriers that make parenting harder for some than others. Faith communities often lead the charge in creating spaces of safety, support, and shared care. That's holy work.

Which of the four Reproductive Justice principles resonates most with your faith values and why?

_____
_____
_____
_____
_____
_____
_____

How have you been taught to make personal decisions in your faith tradition? Have prayer, conscience, or spiritual discernment played a role in how you approach choices about your body?

_____
_____
_____
_____
_____
_____
_____

Have you ever witnessed faith being used to support someone's reproductive decision, rather than judge it? What did that look like?

_____
_____
_____
_____
_____
_____
_____

In what ways can faith communities be stronger allies to people making reproductive decisions?

_____
_____
_____
_____
_____
_____

Centering Faith in the Abortion Debate

Spirituality can be a source of resilience, healing, and ethical clarity. For many, faith provides a framework for loving themselves and others, honoring autonomy, and seeking justice. These are not values that conflict with abortion care—they are the very values that Reproductive Justice is built upon.

The belief that faith and abortion must be at odds comes not from spiritual truth, but from cultural narratives shaped by power, politics, and fear. When we decenter those narratives, we can begin to see the fuller picture: that faith can support us in making thoughtful, loving decisions—even when those decisions include abortion.

"Life Begins at Conception" Is a Theological Belief—Not a Universal Truth

The idea that life begins at conception is not a scientific consensus, nor is it shared across all religions. It is a specific theological belief, rooted primarily in Christian nationalism. Other faith traditions understand the beginning of life differently—some recognize it at birth, others at first breath, and still others have no single position.

For example, according to today's Vatican, life begins at "ensoulment," which current Catholic leadership believes happens at conception. However, through the centuries, Catholics have believed ensoulment happened anywhere from forty days to ninety days after conception, and after 300 years of abortion being legal in the eyes of the church, in 1869 Pope Pius IX declared it illegal from conception, a stance that has stood till this day.[28] Of course, it's estimated that one in four Americans, or 24 percent, who had abortions in 2014 were Catholic,[29] so what church leadership teaches and what people actually do and believe can be quite different. In fact, a 2019 Pew Research poll found that 56 percent of Catholics believed that abortion should be legal in all or most circumstances.[30] As the group Catholics for Choice puts it: "Anti-choice Catholics can be loud, but they are the minority in the church. We believe that the Catholic tradition's teachings on social justice, human dignity, and the primacy of conscience compel us to support the right to reproductive freedom."[31]

Other Christian traditions have put the moment of ensoulment at different times and for different reasons. For much of Christianity, "quickening" was considered the beginning of life, usually around the eighteenth week, and determined by the woman herself. Currently, the official statement from the American Presbyterian Church holds, "We may not know exactly when human life begins." Thus, "When an individual woman faces the decision whether to terminate a pregnancy, the issue is intensely personal and may manifest itself in ways that do not reflect public rhetoric, or do not fit neatly into medical, legal, or policy guidelines. Humans are empowered by the spirit prayerfully to make significant moral choices, including the choice to continue or end a pregnancy."[32] American Baptists state, "Many American Baptists believe that, biblically, human life begins at conception, that abortion is immoral and a destruction of a human being created in God's image (Job 31:15; Psalm 139:13-16; Jeremiah 1:5; Luke 1:44; Proverbs 31:8-9; Galatians 1:15). Many others believe that while abortion is a regrettable reality, it can be a morally acceptable action and they choose to act on the biblical principles of compassion and justice (John 8:1-11; Exodus 21:22-25; Matthew 7:1-5; James 2:2-13) and freedom of will (John 16:13; Roman 14:4-5, 10-13). Many gradations of opinion between these basic positions have been expressed within our fellowship."[33]

I could go on and on through each Christian denomination, and then for the Jewish, Islamic, and Hindu faiths, and do so in my book, *Undue Burden.* The point here is that there is no agreement even within denominations as to when life begins.

Reflection

Given that the timing of when life begins is a diverse theological belief, not a scientific or universally shared truth, how does this diversity—particularly within the Catholic and Presbyterian traditions—challenge or confirm your previous understanding of this topic?

_____
_____
_____
_____
_____
_____
_____
_____
_____
_____

People of Faith Have Abortions

People from all walks of life, including people of faith, have abortions. Some pray before or after their procedures. Some seek counsel from spiritual advisers. Some wrestle deeply; others feel clear and affirmed. Faith doesn't disappear in these moments. It often becomes more present.

By acknowledging the fact that people of faith undertake 60 percent of abortions, we can move the conversation beyond assumptions and toward reality. It allows us to meet people where they are, not where we think they should be.

Reflection

Are you surprised to learn that more than half of abortions in the United States are obtained by people who identify with a faith tradition? Why or why not? How does this information challenge or affirm your understanding of the relationship between faith and abortion? _____

_____

_____

_____

_____

_____

Christian Nationalism Does Not Speak for All Believers

In recent years, the ideology of Christian nationalism has played an outsized role in shaping public narratives around abortion. This movement seeks to merge political power with a narrow interpretation of Christianity, promoting laws that restrict reproductive rights in the name of "religious freedom."

Christian nationalism holds beliefs such as:

- The United States was founded as a Christian nation and should be governed by biblical law
- Christianity deserves privileged status over other religions or belief systems
- Traditional gender roles must be enforced, often positioning women as subservient and motherhood as their primary role
- National identity is tied to religious obedience, with dissent seen as unpatriotic or immoral
- Structural racism is denied or defended, while White Christian identity is often centered as the "true" American identity

But Christian nationalism does not speak for all Christians, and it certainly does not speak for all people of faith. Many religious traditions—including many Christian communities—support reproductive freedom, affirm bodily autonomy, reject racism, and work for justice in healthcare. These perspectives are often drowned out by louder, more extreme voices.

Reflection

How does your personal faith match or differ from the beliefs associated with Christian nationalism? Is there one principle listed above that you agree or disagree with most?

_____
_____
_____
_____
_____

When one religious view becomes law, it violates the core principle of religious freedom and imposes theological beliefs on everyone, regardless of their own spiritual or moral frameworks. Reproductive Justice demands space for multiple beliefs and the freedom for individuals to make decisions aligned with their own values and conscience.

Have you ever experienced a moment when someone's religious beliefs were used to influence or pressure a decision, your own or someone else's? How did that feel, and how did it shape your understanding of the role faith can play in public or personal life?

_____
_____
_____
_____
_____

My Story

For a long time, I kept my spirituality separate from my work. I was raised in the Christian faith. I believe in God. And I understand my values, which are deeply steeped in Christian values. But I also became a physician and an abortion provider, and I know the world doesn't see those things as compatible. The dominant narrative around religion and abortion is full of judgment, and for years, I chose silence. I wasn't ashamed of my faith; I just didn't think there was room for it in the exam room.

That changed one day in my clinic, when a patient preparing for a surgical abortion reached for my hand and asked, "Do you believe in God?" I said yes. "Will you pray with me?" she asked. Without hesitation, I did. She closed her eyes, and we prayed. Her body softened. The room calmed. And the procedure proceeded peacefully.

People of faith have abortions. They wrestle, they pray, they reflect. And they deserve healthcare that honors all of who they are. The idea that Christianity must condemn abortion is a political distortion, not a spiritual truth. I believe, deeply, that faith is not an opponent but an ally. That God trusts us with free will. Supporting someone in making the best decision for their body, their family, and their future is sacred work.

I now speak openly about my Christian faith. I share Bible verses on my personal social media. I tell patients what I believe: that God gives us the power and permission to decide what's best for our bodies, our lives, and our families.

There is a huge, unmet need for spiritual care in abortion spaces. My goal is to make my practice a sanctuary where people can lay down shame and fear and be treated with dignity. This, to me, is the very essence of both good medicine and good faith.

A Shift in Thinking: Faith in Action

In many faith communities, silence from the pro-abortion community has been the norm. Whether out of fear, tradition, or discomfort, conversations often don't happen. Shifting from this passive acceptance of dominant messages to active engagement with the people and places that shape your spiritual life is the first step in supporting the people who need your voice most.

You can choose to show up differently. Whether through a quiet comment, a gesture of support, or a willingness to question what you've always heard, you can be a source of compassion, clarity, and courage.

From Passive to Active

Think of someone you love or worship with who might be struggling with a reproductive decision or has in the past. What do you wish they had heard from their church or family? How might your presence, words, or silence have shaped their experience? What would it mean to be a safe person for someone who shares your faith?

Think through these common scenarios in faith communities. How might you respond in each situation? The first is filled in as an example. Add more scenarios that you've faced.

Situation	Active Faith Practice
Someone shares they're facing an unplanned pregnancy.	Ask gentle questions that open space for conversation.
A congregation member mentions they had an abortion.	
A young person asks about birth control.	
Someone struggles with infertility.	
A family faces a pregnancy with serious complications.	

From Thinking to Action: Joining the Discussion

Here are some common questions that people of faith wrestle with, followed by some gentle, respectful responses that affirm both faith and reproductive freedom:

Question	Brief Response
1. Am I going to hell?	No. God knows your heart. Making a difficult decision with care and conscience is not a rejection of faith.
2. Will God forgive me?	Yes. Many faiths teach that God's love and forgiveness are infinite, even in our hardest choices.
3. Can I still pray after having an abortion?	Absolutely. Your relationship with God remains open and sacred.
4. What will my church community think?	Every community is different, and you are not required to share. Your dignity and privacy matter.
5. Does my religion actually forbid abortion?	Most scriptures don't directly address abortion; interpretations vary widely across and within faiths.
6. Can I still be a good Christian/Muslim/person of faith and work in abortion care?	Yes. Many healthcare providers see their work as an extension of their faith and commitment to justice.
7. How do I tell my religious family?	You don't have to unless it's safe and supportive. Your spiritual well-being comes first.
8. Will I be excommunicated?	Most faiths have no formal process for this. Even where fear exists, policies are often misunderstood.
9. Am I committing murder?	Faith traditions differ on when life begins. Many do not believe personhood starts at conception.

Have you ever had any of the above conversations? How might you expand on any of these responses? Are there any you disagree with?

Your Turn

Most people don't know that people of faith have abortions because, too often, those stories are kept private. The silence reinforces the lie that faith and abortion don't coexist.

Your story has power. Whether it's your own experience or one you witnessed with love and compassion, sharing it helps break the silence. It invites others to feel less alone, and it opens the door to deeper, more honest conversations in our faith communities.

Sharing your story is one of the most important actions you can take to show how faith and abortion care can coexist.

Share a story about when faith and reproductive decision-making intersected in your life or in the life of someone you care about.

- Was it your own decision to have an abortion?
- Did you support a friend or loved one through theirs?
- Did you witness someone struggle—or find peace—because of their faith?
- Was there a moment when your beliefs shifted, deepened, or clarified?

Write about what happened, how faith played a role, and what it meant to you.

_____
_____
_____
_____
_____
_____
_____
_____
_____
_____
_____
_____

Chapter 5 Summary

The assumption that faith and abortion care are incompatible is wrong. We know this because we know that people of faith obtain 60 percent of abortions, and religious traditions hold diverse views on reproductive decisions. The Reproductive Justice framework aligns with core religious values like compassion, dignity, and justice, creating space for believers to support reproductive freedom as an expression of their spiritual convictions rather than a contradiction of them.

While faith can provide moral clarity and support for reproductive decisions, it doesn't exist in isolation from other forces that shape people's experiences. In the next chapter, we'll explore how race, class, and other identities intersect with reproductive healthcare, examining the systemic barriers that make some people's choices easier to access than others.

Room for Thought

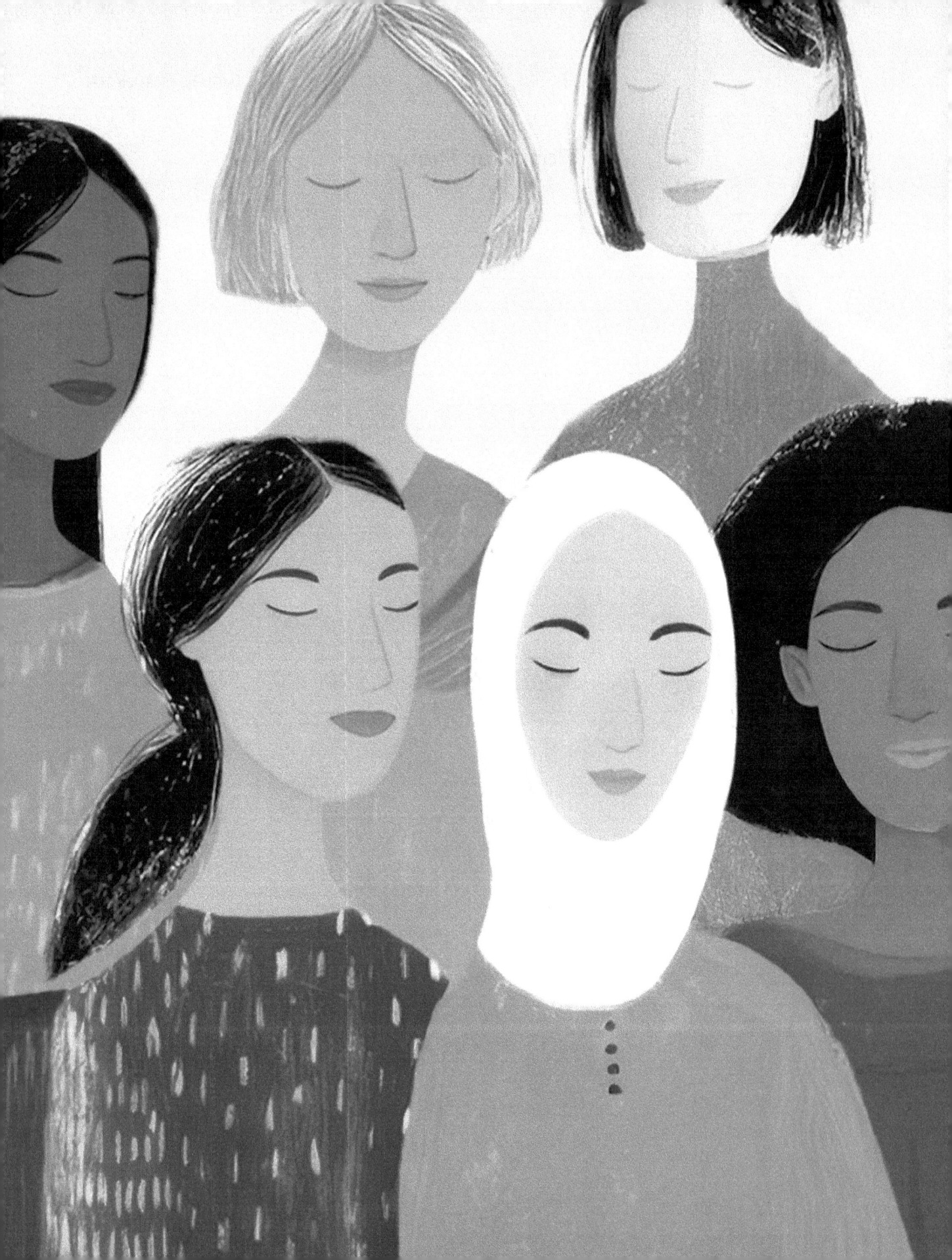

CHAPTER 6

CULTURE, POWER, AND THE FIGHT FOR INCLUSIVE CARE

> Who has access to safe, affirming healthcare, and who is denied it?

Why This Question?

We all play a role in who has access to care and who doesn't. We participate in systems—even if unintentionally—that create barriers to inclusive care for ourselves and others. Only when we acknowledge this can we take steps to ensure inclusion for everyone.

Systems are built on cultural assumptions and biases. Examining these biases isn't meant to shame anyone. We all have unconscious biases. Instead, the goal is to examine them honestly, so we can see how they perpetuate unjust systems. We can create an environment where people can

BEYOND CHOICE

bring their true selves to every healthcare encounter. We can lay the foundation for inclusive and equitable care. But first, we have to look at the systems that exist and our roles within them.

So, I ask: **Who has access to safe, affirming healthcare, and who is denied it?**

Have you ever felt as if you had to hide parts of your identity or change how you spoke or dressed before a medical appointment? If so, what made you feel that way?

_____
_____
_____
_____
_____
_____
_____
_____
_____

Have you ever held back from bringing up a specific health concern with a provider because you worried about being judged or dismissed?

_____
_____
_____
_____
_____
_____
_____
_____
_____

Do you think it's easier for some people to be their authentic selves in healthcare settings than it is for you? Which friends, family members, or others in your community might find it harder or easier? What accounts for the difference?

_____
_____
_____
_____
_____
_____
_____
_____
_____
_____

Our Shared Experience

Recently, I saw two adults who appeared to have Down syndrome holding hands, clearly in a romantic relationship. My first thought was, *How cute—boyfriend and girlfriend*. It felt like a positive reaction.

But later, I realized that my need to comment on their relationship revealed my internalized judgment that their relationship wasn't normal. Labeling a romantic relationship between two people with Down syndrome as "cute" can inadvertently lead to substandard care.

How Cultural Assumptions About Intellectual Disability Affect Care

Underlying Assumption	Barrier to Care
People with intellectual disabilities are asexual	Sexual disease testing or pregnancy tests overlooked
They cannot understand or benefit from discussions about sex and relationships	Inadequate sexual education, contributing to unwanted pregnancy or sexual harassment
They are not seen as needing or capable of making reproductive choices	Contraceptive needs often overlooked
They shouldn't have children	Coercive counseling around sterilization and long-term contraception
They are unfit to be parents	Limited access to fertility support services

Question for Reflection

Have you ever made assumptions about someone because of their disability, race, socioeconomic status, gender, sexual orientation, or other cultural aspects? Here are some examples. Fill in the table with your experiences:

Example Thought	Underlying Assumption	Barrier to Reproductive Healthcare
"Black women are so strong. They can get through anything."	Black women don't need emotional or physical support.	Pain and symptoms may be dismissed; less likely to be offered support after pregnancy loss.
"Gay people don't need to worry about reproductive health."	LGBTQIA people aren't involved in reproduction.	Lack of inclusive conversations about fertility procedures, surrogacy, or co-parenting.
"There are other healthcare providers who will care for gay and transgender patients even if I don't."	Denying care based on your beliefs or morals is a neutral decision.	Inability to find a care provider that's close enough or affordable.
"She's Catholic. She probably isn't interested in abortion care."	Cultural identity is linked with healthcare desires.	Default to pro-natal care; limited support for contraception or abortion.
"She's undocumented. She probably wants the cheapest solution to her problem."	Immigration or economic status aligns with healthcare decisions.	Providers may withhold information, assuming patients can't or won't access care.

Reflection Question

Have you ever had one of these assumptions applied to you or found yourself making a similar assumption about someone else? What was the impact? _____

_____
_____
_____
_____
_____
_____
_____

Our Shared Values

Whether we realize it or not, each of us has been taught a set of values about what a family should look like, who deserves care, and who gets left behind. These values are not neutral. They are shaped by culture and reinforced by systems of power that center certain identities while marginalizing others. White supremacy, patriarchy, ableism, fundamentalist Christianity, and heteronormativity don't just live in laws and policies. They live in us.

DID YOU KNOW?

Culture goes far beyond food, holidays, and traditions. It's the invisible framework that shapes our deepest assumptions about what constitutes so-called normal behavior. Culture is actively shaped by systems of power, and we often carry and act on these learned beliefs without realizing it, feeling uncomfortable with anything outside the perceived norm, often based on others' (or our own!) appearance or identity.

We carry our cultural values into every interaction, including healthcare encounters. And often, we act on them without realizing it. Maybe we feel discomfort when someone uses a pronoun we're not used to. Maybe we think, even subconsciously, that disabled people shouldn't be parents, or that certain families are more legitimate than others. These aren't just personal feelings. They're learned beliefs, passed down by a system that benefits from keeping some people on the margins.

You may have been harmed by these values. You may also have upheld them. Most of us have done both.

It's often hard to look honestly at what you've been taught.

Check the box that most reflects your honest response:

Cultural Values About Healthcare Access	I Agree With This	I Disagree With This	I'm Not Sure
It bothers me that I have to include my pronouns on an intake form in my doctor's office.			
There may be situations in which people with disabilities probably shouldn't have children.			
Traditional families (man, woman, children) are more stable and thus best for children.			
If someone can't afford reproductive care, they shouldn't get pregnant.			
Personal details—like gender identity or sexual orientation—aren't usually necessary to share in a healthcare setting.			
Some communities seem to face more problems due to the choices they make.			
People who don't speak English shouldn't expect healthcare workers to accommodate them.			
It's ridiculous to have to say, "birthing people" instead of just saying "women."			
A birth worker should be able to choose not to work with transgender clients if it makes them uncomfortable.			
People experiencing homelessness probably can't handle the responsibility of having children.			

Did any of your values surprise you when you saw them written out? _____

_____
_____
_____
_____
_____

Can you think of a specific time when one of these values influenced how you treated someone or how you expected to be treated in a healthcare setting? _____

_____
_____
_____
_____
_____

New Thinking: How Culture Shapes Healthcare Access

Accessing healthcare in America isn't easy. Accessing healthcare when you are outside the dominant paradigm can be close to impossible. But why would anyone want to deny a person healthcare? What good is there in harming others? In making their lives difficult, if not impossible?

A racist, patriarchal society has an interest in upholding its vision of a society in which the people who have been pushed to the margins "rightly" suffer. We are taught to punish those who "deserve their fate" by not conforming to the perceived norm. When society puts people "in their place," it creates a cycle of misery. The conservative image of a heteronormative, Christian, White family can only be upheld when anyone who defies it suffers. Then, we blame individuals, and the cycle continues.

Consider LGBTQIA individuals. It is legal in most states for private healthcare providers to turn away LGBTQIA patients for personal, religious, or moral objections. This leaves them with fewer healthcare options. Then, when abortion is banned, accessible reproductive health clinics close, and doctors move away, limiting choice even more. Due to abortion bans:

- 11 percent of LGBTQIA people were forced to change medical providers or struggled to find them, compared to 2 percent of non-LGBTQIA adults.[34]

When we look at intersectional aspects of access to care, the picture is even starker:

- 15 percent of Black LGBTQIA people had to travel out of state to access reproductive healthcare compared to 1 percent of non-LGBTQIA people.[35]

I have received patient referrals from physicians who tell me how relieved they are that I provide abortion or gender-affirming hormone therapy because they don't "feel comfortable" addressing that part of care. For LGBTQIA individuals, if they can't find a provider like me who's "comfortable," issues arise, such as being called the wrong pronouns or being deadnamed—called their legal name, instead of the name they go by. This is incredibly traumatizing, and they often just stop seeking care completely.

Reflection Question

Imagine going to a doctor who isn't comfortable with you. Or, recall an experience where this actually happened to you or someone you love. How did it feel?

My Story

In my clinical work and in some professional spaces, I have encountered significant resistance to asking for and using people's preferred pronouns. Transphobia is pervasive.

When I hear women's health practitioners say, "I'm not going to work with trans men," I'll ask, "Why not?"

We can't assume that pregnancy or abortion care is strictly a woman's issue. Transgender men and nonbinary people can become pregnant and also need care. When considering the lack of abortion care available, we must imagine being a transgender man forced to carry a pregnancy to term, an experience that fundamentally conflicts with their sense of self. That's medical trauma.

Practitioners must examine the source of their discomfort and understand why it holds such significance for them. Their role is literally to help a pregnant person through prenatal care, birth, and the immediate postpartum period. Why do they care so much about what their pronouns are or how they'll chestfeed their baby? There has to be more reflection.

When I first decided to expand my practice to include gender-affirming care, I needed to fundamentally transform how I treated my patients, starting with the forms they filled out during intake. I began by updating our standard forms in our electronic health records to include sexual orientation and gender identity (SOGI) data. For example, I collected pronouns and revised the general female history section to say, "If you have a uterus, continue." I also changed the language to "Have you ever chestfed?" instead of breastfed. This signaled to people that this was a safe space.

What happened next surprised me, but it shouldn't have.

Two patients particularly stand out in my memory. One established patient, who came in for a routine wellness exam, said, "Dr. Taylor, I was so happy to see you offer gender-affirming hormone therapy. I've been wanting to transition. I'm hoping you can get me started." It was the first time she'd ever shared that desire with me. Another established patient told me she was considering transitioning but wasn't sure. I have a process for exploring dysphoria, the deep sense of discomfort or distress that may arise when someone's gender identity doesn't align with the sex they were assigned at birth. We worked through it together, and she ultimately decided it wasn't the right path for her.

In both cases, these individuals needed to feel safe and supported before they could even begin the conversation. Technically, they always had access to care, but without comfort and trust, they couldn't make use of it in a meaningful or informed way.

When we, as providers, make a deliberate choice to be inclusive, we can better serve all our patients without leaving anyone behind. It was the way I presented and collected information that let people know I would honor their authentic selves. Once they sensed I was on their side, our interactions completely changed. Although providers are often hesitant to ask patients about sexual preference due to concerns about embarrassment, research shows that most patients do not share this fear. In fact, a straightforward, open question on registration forms, such as "Do you have sex with men, women, or both?" can provide physicians with important information and foster communication channels that may prove essential in understanding and addressing health needs.[36]

Inclusion isn't easy. It must be intentional. At first, I had to encourage my staff to ensure everyone was asked all the questions consistently. If the patient didn't answer on the form, they had to ask. That was a learning curve for my team. When we collect SOGI data universally, we remove the burden from individual patients to out themselves and advocate for inclusive care. We make inclusion the default rather than the exception.

A Shift in Thinking: Culture, Power, and Inclusive Care

The systems that exclude people from healthcare didn't emerge from nowhere. They were deliberately constructed by those who benefit from keeping certain groups marginalized. White supremacy, patriarchy, and fundamentalist Christianity are the power structures that have shaped the traditional idea of family: how women and men are supposed to behave, how families are supposed to look, and how children should be raised.

When we make judgments about who deserves care and who doesn't—based on someone's sexual orientation, gender identity, race, socioeconomic situation, or ethnicity—we're participating in the oppression passed down by those who built and benefit from these structures. White supremacy and patriarchy laid the foundation. But we're the ones keeping it going in our interactions with one another. They started it, but they no longer have to take any action. The seeds were planted. Now we water them ourselves with our judgment and actions.

Reflection Question

Access to abortion care is perhaps the starkest example of how systems are set up to grant care to those with "acceptable" identities—those who are White, wealthy, cisgender, heterosexual, or married—while denying or restricting access for those who are seen as "unacceptable." What does this say about whose lives, families, and choices are valued in our society—and whose are not?

_____

_____

_____

_____

_____

_____

_____

From Thinking to Action: Expanding Access to Care

Understanding how culture and power shape healthcare access is only the beginning. Real change happens when we translate this awareness into concrete action that challenges exclusion and creates more inclusive spaces for everyone who needs care.

Reflection Questions

Personal Experience: Now that you've thought about your values deeply, can you identify judgments you made about who deserves care?

_____

_____

_____

_____

_____

_____

Emotional Response: What did you feel when you read about or experienced how people are excluded from the healthcare system? How might these feelings guide your actions moving forward?

Knowledge and Skills: What unique knowledge, skills, or resources do you possess that might be valuable in creating more inclusive healthcare environments? For example, are you a healthcare provider who could change intake forms? A community leader who could advocate for inclusive policies? Someone with lived experience who could educate healthcare providers?

Community Need: In your community, which groups fall outside the dominant White, heteronormative, fundamentalist Christian paradigm? Do you have intersections with any of these groups?

Existing Movements: Are you already involved in social justice movements that intersect with healthcare access? How might your current activism connect to fighting for inclusive care? What new connections could you build between different advocacy groups?

Personal Values: Which of your cultural assumptions about who deserves care have been most challenged by this chapter? How does confronting these beliefs align with your core values about human dignity and justice?

_____
_____
_____
_____
_____
_____

Impact Assessment: Where do you believe your contribution could make the greatest difference in creating more inclusive healthcare? Consider both the need and your capacity to effect change—whether that's in your family, workplace, community, or broader advocacy efforts.

_____
_____
_____
_____
_____
_____

Your Turn

Culture responds to oppression in powerful ways. People build culture to survive and thrive under oppressive systems. When the power structure tries to dismantle protections, people still find joy, still build community, and still celebrate.

Think about the 2025 Met Gala, where Black excellence took center stage with the theme of Black dandyism. It became a cultural rebellion when people of all backgrounds joined in, centering the marginalized and making it the accepted mode of being. It was a community-wide celebration that centered joy, instead of trauma. This is a prime example of culture rising in direct opposition to systems designed to exclude and diminish. It's powerful because it reclaims space and redefines what's possible.

Even in bleak scenarios, culture and subcultures continue to thrive. Groups are still finding joy. And in that joy, they bring themselves back into the conversation, forcing people to confront their existence. Culture becomes a force for healing and justice, rather than exclusion.

Acting on Joy

In Your Personal Life: What small acts of resistance could you embrace? How might you model inclusive behavior that signals safety to others who might feel excluded?

In Your Community: How can you support or amplify cultural celebrations and spaces that center marginalized voices? What events, organizations, or initiatives could use your participation or resources?

In Your Networks: How might you use your social media, workplace conversations, or family gatherings to uplift stories and perspectives that challenge dominant cultural narratives about who deserves care and belonging?

Circle at least six actions you're going to take in the next week, month, and year. Add your own if you can:

Who Is Being Denied Care	Ally (Interpersonal)	Advocate (Institutional/Professiona)	Activist (Systemic/Public)
A transgender person denied gender-affirming care	Respect names/pronouns and challenge transphobic comments in your circles.	Push for inclusive healthcare policies in your workplace, school, or community.	Join or support efforts to overturn laws that ban gender-affirming care.
A Black woman facing medical racism during pregnancy	Listen without judgment and validate her experience.	Work to ensure implicit bias training is actually implemented in your clinic/hospital/place of worship.	Support legislation for maternal health equity and fund Black-led birth justice organizations.
A person with an intellectual disability is excluded from reproductive health education	Use accessible language and include them in conversations about relationships and health.	Advocate for inclusive sex ed programs at your school or organization.	Campaign for disability-inclusive healthcare laws and public health materials.
A person with low income, unable to travel for abortion care	Help them research local resources and support without shame.	Push for flexible policies (like paid leave or transportation support) at your workplace.	Donate to or volunteer with abortion funds and Reproductive Justice orgs fighting for policy change.
A queer teen shamed by a school counselor for asking about birth control	Affirm their right to accurate information and offer resources.	Push your school or district to adopt LGBTQIA-inclusive curricula.	Show up at school board meetings to oppose harmful abstinence-only or religiously biased education.

Chapter 6 Summary

Systems of culture, power, and oppression shape healthcare access, and we must move beyond individual prejudices to understand the structural forces that exclude certain people from care. These systems were deliberately constructed by those who benefit from keeping certain groups marginalized, and we often unconsciously participate in maintaining these barriers through our judgments about who deserves care.

Cultural resistance matters. Communities can come together to build joy, celebration, and authentic expression even under oppressive conditions, and this helps open doors to people who need care.

The work ahead starts with dismantling harmful assumptions and then actively creating inclusive spaces. By recognizing our role in either perpetuating or challenging exclusion, we can begin to transform healthcare environments into places where everyone can bring their authentic selves and receive the care they deserve.

In the next chapter, we'll explore how to sustain this work for the long term, building movements that can weather setbacks and continue fighting for inclusive care across generations.

Room for Thought

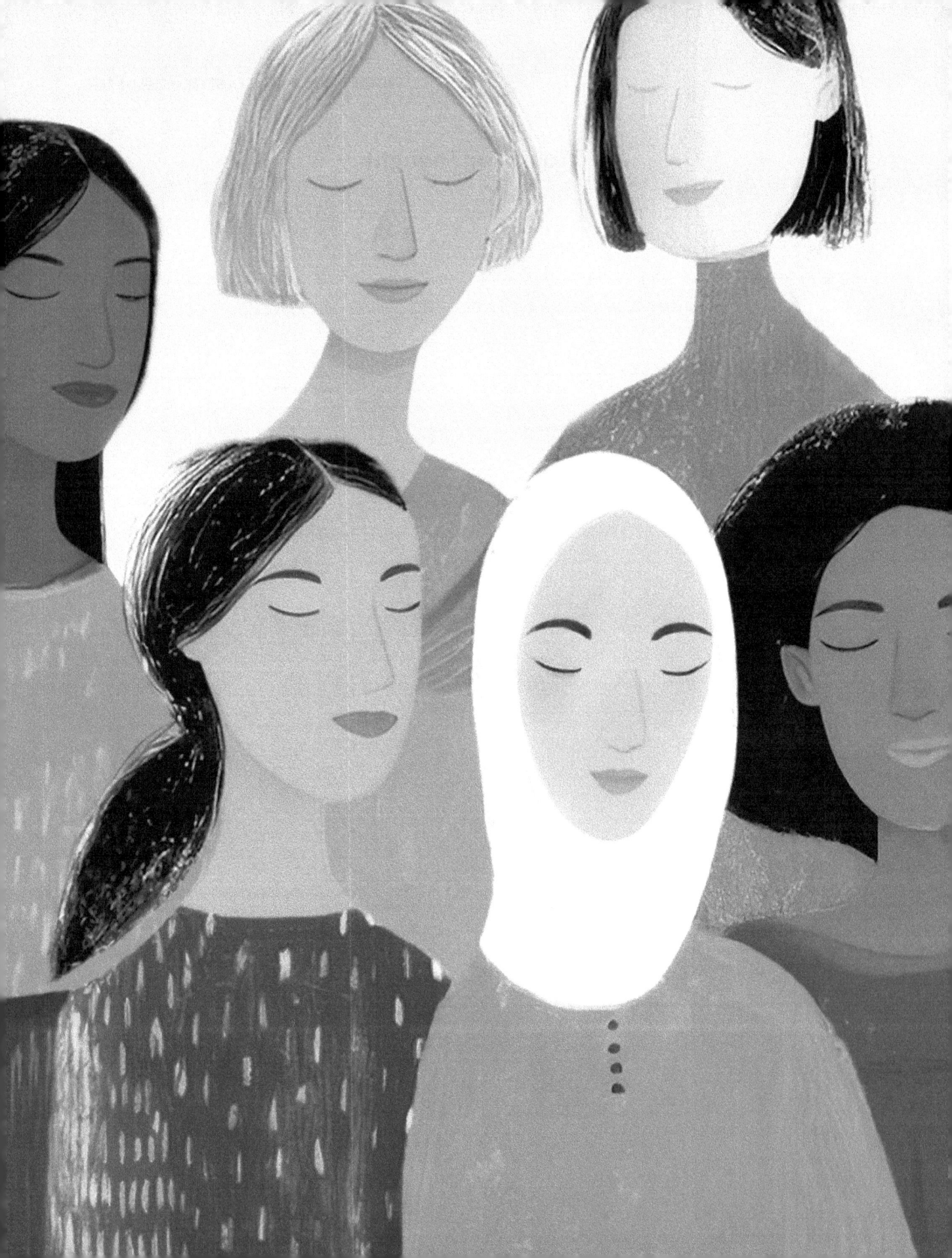

CHAPTER 7

KEEPING THE MOVEMENT ALIVE

> How will you sustain your commitment to Reproductive Justice for yourself, your community, and the generations to come?

Why This Question?

Learning doesn't lead to transformation. People lose 80 percent of what they read. More often, suffering leads to wisdom, and through wisdom, we are transformed.

$$\text{Suffering} \rightarrow \text{Wisdom} \rightarrow \text{Transformation}$$

Some of you have experienced the pain and trauma we have worked through in this book, and some of you have not. Yet, through participating in the work of this workbook, you've undertaken the practice of deliberative transformation, which is the process of true change without suffering. This comes from intentional, sustained efforts toward personal growth—learning, reflecting, and acting with purpose over time.

Examining Current Values → Learning New Values → Acting on Those Values → Transformation

In picking up this book and making it to the end, you have decided that you aren't going to wait for moments of suffering to push you to evolve. From now on, you will consistently wake yourself up and consciously move forward.

Transformation is a perspective shift. A mind expanded doesn't shrink back. But the process must be continuous, so you keep moving forward.

So, I ask: **How will you sustain your commitment to Reproductive Justice for yourself, your community, and the generations to come?**

As you think about your own experiences with causes you've cared about, what patterns do you notice in how your commitments have waxed and waned over time?

Whether you're new to Reproductive Justice work or have been engaged for years, the challenge is the same: How do you keep going? Based on your previous experiences with working for causes, what advice would you give yourself for staying with it?

_____
_____
_____
_____
_____
_____
_____
_____
_____
_____

Question for Thought

Is it possible that when you close this book, you will stop paying attention to Reproductive Justice issues? What barriers to continuing might stand in your way?

_____
_____
_____
_____
_____
_____
_____
_____
_____

Our Shared Experience

In my experience as a Reproductive Justice advocate and coalition builder, I've witnessed a predictable pattern: People begin this work with passion and determination, but many struggle to sustain their commitment when the reality of long-term advocacy sets in.

When I ask advocates and activists about their experiences with sustaining movement work, these are some of the responses I often hear:

Common Experiences with Losing Momentum and Movement Fatigue:

- "I was fired up after that rally, but then what?"
- "I started following more news, but it became overwhelming."
- "My friends got tired of hearing me talk about reproductive rights."
- "The work felt too big for one person to make a difference."
- "I got busy with my life, and the urgency faded."
- "I feel like I'm constantly fighting and nothing changes."
- "I'm tired of being the only one who seems to care in my community."
- "I burned out trying to do everything."

Common Experiences of Those Who Sustain Their Commitment:

- "I found my specific lane and focused my energy there."
- "I connected with others who share this commitment."
- "I learned to celebrate small wins along the way."
- "I made self-care part of my activism."
- "I accepted that I won't see all the change in my lifetime, but my children might."

Reflection Exercise

Think about the statements above. Which ones feel familiar to your own experience with sustaining commitment to causes you care about? What patterns do you notice in yourself?

_____
_____
_____
_____
_____
_____
_____
_____
_____
_____

Our Shared Values

The challenges of doing the work that needs to be done often persist because of deeply ingrained values we learned about commitment, activism, and sustainability. These values shape how we approach long-term work and determine whether we can sustain our efforts over time. Do you recognize any of the values listed below in yourself?

Values About Sustaining Commitment

My Values	YES, I Hold This Value	NO, I Don't Hold This Value	Unsure...
Passion alone can sustain me.			
Good people keep fighting, no matter what.			
If I really care, I'll always put the work first.			
Taking time for myself can wait when others are suffering.			
I'm strong; I can handle anything.			
Asking for help shows weakness.			
Sometimes, I need to do everything myself.			
If I can't see immediate results, I'm not happy.			
My worth is measured by how much I sacrifice.			
If it's important, it won't feel hard.			
Celebration is frivolous when there's still work to do.			

Reflection Exercise

Look back at your values. Did any of these contribute to your experiences with losing momentum or burning out when working in a movement?

_____
_____
_____
_____
_____
_____

New Thinking: Five Strategies for Sustainable Advocacy

I've learned that the values I held about commitment and activism were actually setting me up to burn out. But there's another way. During my time facilitating reproductive rights and justice coalition spaces since 2019, and through my own experiences with burnout and ongoing recovery, I've developed five strategies that challenge conventional thinking about what it means to be committed to this work.

These strategies may initially feel uncomfortable. They challenge much of what we've been taught about dedication and sacrifice. But they represent a sustainable approach to advocacy that can help you stay engaged for the long haul.

1. Prioritize Well-being and Mental Health

Old thinking: Good advocates sacrifice themselves for the cause.
New thinking: Self-care is not selfish.

As Audre Lorde famously stated, "Caring for myself is not self-indulgence, it is self-preservation—and that is an act of political warfare." Lorde's radical vision challenges the notion of self-care as luxury, framing it instead as critical defiance against systems that demand constant productivity and self-sacrifice, particularly from members of marginalized communities.

Practical Steps:

- **Self-Care Is Not Selfish:** In times of stress, it's crucial to actively engage in practices that support your mental and emotional health. This could include spending time in nature, connecting with loved ones, engaging in hobbies, or seeking professional support if needed. Burnout is a significant risk during prolonged periods of political tension.
- **Limit News Consumption**: While staying informed is important, constant exposure to distressing news can be overwhelming. Set boundaries for how and when you consume news, and seek out diverse, reputable sources rather than being caught in doomscrolling.
- **Find Your Community**: Connect with others who share your concerns and values. Mutual support systems are vital for emotional resilience and can provide a sense of solidarity and shared purpose. Sometimes, this can be an in-real-life group. Other times, it might be online or virtual. For example, an app is in development as a companion to this book to provide forums for like-minded individuals.

2. Strengthen Community and Mutual Aid Networks

Old thinking: Real activism means total sacrifice, often in competition with others, until a visible win is achieved.

New thinking: Strong local networks provide a buffer against external pressures and sustain the movement.

- **Build Local Resilience:** Focus on strengthening local community ties. This could involve organizing mutual aid networks, sharing resources, creating skill-sharing groups, or simply getting to know your neighbors better.
- **Support Grassroots Organizations:** Invest your time, energy, or resources in grassroots organizations that are working directly to support affected communities and protect civil liberties. These groups often have the most direct impact on the ground.
- **Share Information and Skills:** Knowledge is power. Share accurate information, practical skills (e.g., first aid, legal rights, community organizing), and resources within your trusted networks. Don't just show up to receive—disseminate!

3. Understand and Protect Your Rights

Old thinking: Someone else will handle the legal stuff.
New thinking: Knowledge is power, and understanding your rights strengthens the entire movement.

- **Know Your Rights:** Familiarize yourself with your civil liberties and legal rights. Organizations like the American Civil Liberties Union and local legal aid groups often provide resources and training on how to respond to various challenges to your rights. The Center for Reproductive Rights and the National Women's Law Center are two other excellent resources.
- **Document and Report:** If you experience or witness civil liberties violations, document them thoroughly (date, time, location, details of what happened, witnesses) and report them to relevant organizations. This data is crucial for advocacy and legal challenges.
- **Support Legal Advocacy:** Support organizations that are engaged in legal challenges to restrictive policies. Litigation can be a powerful tool to push back against harmful executive orders and legislation.

4. Engage in Strategic Advocacy and Activism

Old thinking: My work on a single issue won't matter enough to make a difference.
New thinking: Focus on impact rather than trying to do everything.

- **Focus on Impact:** Identify key issues where your efforts can have the most impact. For reproductive health, this might include advocating for equitable access to contraception, comprehensive sex education, or addressing maternal mortality. Find your lane!
- **Coalition Building:** Work across different groups and movements. Building broad coalitions strengthens collective power and amplifies voices, especially for marginalized communities who may face unique intersectional challenges. Pull in neighbors, classmates, and church groups.
- **Civic Engagement (Even When Challenging):** Continue to participate in democratic processes as much as possible, including voting, advocating for fair elections, and holding

elected officials accountable. Even in challenging times, these avenues can still offer opportunities for change. Do it!

5. Cultivate Hope and Long-Term Vision

Old thinking: Incremental change is the way. We can't ask for too much too soon.
New thinking: Progress happens on a long arc. Small victories matter, but should be part of a long-term vision.

- **Remember History:** Recognize that periods of intense political challenge are not new. History offers lessons in resilience, resistance, and eventual progress. Understand the long arc of civil rights and social justice movements.
- **Celebrate Small Victories:** Acknowledge and celebrate small wins. This helps to sustain morale and reminds us that progress, however incremental, is possible.
- **Maintain Your Vision:** Hold onto a clear vision of the just and equitable society you are striving for. This long-term perspective can provide motivation and direction during difficult times.

Survival in challenging times isn't about passive endurance. It's about active resilience, collective action, and unwavering commitment to principles of justice and human dignity.

Which of these five strategies feels most challenging to you personally? Why do you think that is? _____
_____
_____
_____
_____
_____

Which strategy do you think would make the biggest difference in your ability to sustain your commitment to Reproductive Justice? _____

_____
_____
_____
_____
_____
_____

My Story

I've always worked to be the best version of myself. That's just the way I approach life. But what I've learned through years of Reproductive Justice work is that sustainable advocacy requires more than individual transformation. It demands an understanding that growth happens in relationship with others and that lasting change requires building coalitions, even when they don't unfold as planned.

Over the past several years, I've helped launch multiple coalitions: some faltered, some evolved, and two remain active as originally formed as of the writing of this book. Each experience has taught me something new about leadership, community, and the importance of sustainability.

When I first became involved in Reproductive Justice advocacy, I looked for a Reproductive Justice coalition in Arizona, and couldn't find one. So I made myself available. A group had received funding to start a coalition. I attended a couple of meetings, and then it was over suddenly. The coalition disbanded.

After that, I wrote a grant. I didn't get funded, but I stayed in touch with the funder. Eventually, they gave me seed funding and paired me with someone else to start a coalition. We gave it our best shot, but because the partnership hadn't formed organically, it never truly clicked. I left, and many others did too.

Then I was asked to start an all-Black coalition. At first, I said no. It's a lot of work. When you start something, you're accountable for making it succeed. You hope others will share the load, but that doesn't always happen.

But I reconsidered. That group still exists today: the Empower Alliance for Reproductive Justice. Progress has proceeded at an intentional and steady pace.

Later, there was another attempt to form a BIPOC Reproductive Justice coalition, which became inactive after a couple of years. The final Reproductive Justice coalition I was involved in forming came out of a broader reproductive rights coalition that disbanded. The Arizona Proactive Reproductive Justice Alliance is a group of grassroots organizations and individual activists across Arizona working in partnership with national organizations. We drafted a sweeping abortion restrictions repeal bill that was introduced during the 2025 Arizona legislative session. Although the bill did not get a committee hearing, we celebrated this enormous feat of drafting and having the bill introduced. We worked two years toward that goal.

In the end, I've launched coalitions that failed, coalitions that evolved, and coalitions that endured—but all of them taught me something. You have to be committed to making it work. You must nurture relationships, recruit talent, and hope that others will be inspired to carry the work forward.

For me, the key is continuing the projects that bring me joy and that have the potential to make real, lasting change in people's lives.

In doing this work, I've had important realizations. One is that I carry so much that when I step away, there's a real risk that things won't get done. I had to shift my mindset and accept that. I had to clarify what truly matters: what absolutely needs to be done, and what can wait. If some things fall through the cracks, it'll be okay, and I'll be okay. Getting to that point took time.

Learning to take breaks was part of that evolution. While writing this book, I took a seven-day cruise through the Eastern Caribbean during the summer. I wrote on LinkedIn afterward:

> *As a Black woman leading health justice organizations that operate at the intersection of medical practice, social justice, and systemic challenges, the concept of rest as resistance is not merely theoretical—it's acutely necessary.*

That time away was about resisting burnout, reclaiming well-being, and finding empowerment through rest. In a world that often seeks to diminish or erase the needs of those fighting for justice, choosing rest is a radical assertion of worth and a strategic move to ensure longevity in our work.

The sustainability strategies I've shared with you stem from years of trial and error, including coalition building, burnout, and hard-won clarity about what it takes to make a difference.

A Shift in Thinking: Your Advocacy Journey

Transform your thinking about what it means to be committed to Reproductive Justice:

Old Unsustainable Values	New Sustainable Values
Passion alone will sustain me.	Passion plus practical strategies sustain me.
Good advocates never need breaks.	Good advocates take intentional breaks to preserve their capacity.
I should work constantly if I care.	Strategic work with boundaries is more effective than constant work.
Self-care is selfish when others suffer.	Self-care is an act of political resistance and preservation.
I should be able to handle what comes.	Asking for support strengthens both me and the movement.
I am more successful when doing everything myself.	Success means building collective power.
If I can't see immediate results, I'm not effective.	Change happens on a long arc; small victories matter.
My worth is measured by sacrifice.	My worth comes from sustained, strategic contribution.
Individual action is most important.	Collective action creates lasting change.
I must be involved in everything.	Focus and specialization create a greater impact.

Reflection Exercise

Which old value do you find hardest to let go of? Why do you think it's difficult to release?

_____
_____
_____
_____
_____
_____
_____

Which new value excites you most? How might adopting this perspective change your approach to Reproductive Justice work? _____

_____
_____
_____
_____
_____
_____
_____
_____

From Thinking to Action: Sustaining Your Commitment

Now that you understand both the obstacles to sustaining advocacy work and the strategies that can help you stay engaged, it's time to create your personal sustainability plan.

Reflection Questions

Personal Experience: As you think about your past efforts to stay committed to causes you care about, which of the five sustainability strategies would have been most helpful? Which do you most need to develop now?

Emotional Response: Which part of this chapter made you feel most hopeful about your ability to sustain your commitment? Which part felt most challenging or overwhelming?

Knowledge and Skills: What unique strengths do you bring to Reproductive Justice work that could help you sustain your engagement? (For example: Are you good at building relationships? Do you have experience with strategic planning? Are you skilled at self-care practices?) _____

_____

_____

_____

_____

_____

Community Need: In your specific community, what community groups can you align with so that you're not fighting the fight alone? _____

_____

_____

_____

_____

_____

Existing Movements: What movements already exist, so you can join them, instead of going it alone? _____

_____

_____

_____

_____

_____

Personal Values: Do you think you can make self-care one of your most important values? If not, what changes are needed to get you there? _____

_____
_____
_____
_____
_____
_____
_____

Impact Assessment: What is one thing you want to achieve that you can focus on for years or even decades? _____

_____
_____
_____
_____
_____
_____
_____

Your Turn: Your Sustainability Action Plan

Based on your reflections, create a concrete plan for sustaining your commitment to Reproductive Justice:

Strategy 1: Well-being and Mental Health

What is one specific practice you will adopt to support your mental and emotional health?

Strategy 2: Community and Mutual Aid

Who are two to three people you can connect with who share your commitment to this work?

Strategy 3: Understanding Your Rights

What is one way you will deepen your knowledge of your rights or those of your community? _____

Strategy 4: Strategic Advocacy

What is your lane in Reproductive Justice work? Where will you focus your efforts for maximum impact? _____

Strategy 5: Hope and Long-term Vision

How will you celebrate small victories? What practices will help you maintain your long-term vision?

Your Commitment Statement

Draft a personal commitment statement that captures how you will sustain your engagement with Reproductive Justice:

I commit to sustaining my work in Reproductive Justice by taking care of myself. To maintain my capacity for this work, I will…

I understand this is long-term work, so I commit to staying engaged even when progress feels slow. I am motivated to continue because…

Setting Actionable Goals

Based on your reflections, set at least three concrete actions you'll take in the next three months to build your sustainability practices:

This month, I will:

Next month, I will:

In three months, I will:

To stay accountable, I will:

When I face challenges, I will:

_____

_____

_____

_____

_____

_____

_____

Chapter 7 Summary

Sustainable advocacy is about showing up consistently, taking care of yourself and your community, and keeping your eyes on the long-term vision of justice. Your sustained commitment, however it looks, is needed for the movement and for the generations to come.

Room for Thought

CONCLUSION

THE WORK IS NOW

On September 30, 2025, just after midnight, approximately 100 heavily armed federal agents representing ICE, US Border Patrol, the FBI, and the Bureau of Alcohol, Tobacco, Firearms, and Explosives (ATF) descended before dawn on a 130-unit apartment complex in Chicago's South Shore neighborhood. Arriving in military-style vehicles and dropping onto the roof from a Black Hawk helicopter, the agents forcefully entered the building and broke down residents' doors. They zip-tied and detained almost every resident of the building, most of whom were pulled from their beds, including dozens of Black Americans and their children, and kept them handcuffed outside on the street for hours, regardless of citizenship status.

They separated zip-tied children—some zip-tied to one another—from their zip-tied parents.

Eventually, most residents were let go. Thirty-seven arrests were made, including undocumented immigrants and US citizens.

This was not abstract political maneuvering. It was the physical, visceral denial of the first and fourth tenets of Reproductive Justice: the right to bodily autonomy and the right to raise our children in a safe and healthy environment. That night, America unapologetically used full military force to deny the fundamental rights and security of marginalized groups, sending a clear message that the state reserves the right to terrorize Black and immigrant families within its own borders.

When the plan for this workbook was drafted in early 2025, we spoke of a gathering storm. We spoke of a world beyond Roe, where our fight for reproductive freedom would have to move beyond choice to embrace the full, radical vision of Reproductive Justice. We knew the fight was not just for the right *not* to have children, but also for the right to have children and to nurture the children we have in a safe and healthy environment.

Today, as you close this book, we must acknowledge that the storm is no longer approaching—it has broken. The terrifying political shift we were preparing for has arrived with brutal clarity.

So much has changed since we began this journey, and the work you have done—examining your personal participation in oppressive systems, connecting your personal experience to the political, and creating a plan for sustained commitment—is no longer preparatory. It is for immediate use.

This urgency is defined by the indelible images of the mayhem that was unleashed on the people of South Shore Chicago. When armed agents can invade the sanctuary of 130 homes, detain Black and Brown Americans, and bind children and their parents, the state is making an unambiguous statement about whose bodily autonomy and safety are disposable. This horrific event is the final, terrifying proof of the systems of reproductive oppression we have been analyzing in these pages. The same forces that target Black women for pregnancy loss, as in the Brittany Watts story, and use state funds to investigate and remove children from poor families, have fully militarized.

For me, as a Black woman physician and activist, this moment compels me to share my deepest thought: We can no longer afford to be passive participants in an oppressive system. The system is not broken; it is functioning exactly as it was designed to deny Black, Indigenous, and marginalized communities the right to survive and thrive.

Your completed workbook is now a blueprint for active survival and sustained resistance.

You have found your voice and identified your lane. Now, you must integrate your new values, such as moving from the individual right to privacy to collective human rights and community well-being. These values must be embedded into every action you take.

The survival of our communities depends on transforming the grief and outrage from events like the raid in Chicago into an unwavering commitment to protect our people.

Close this book, but keep its lessons in your hands, your heart, and your community. The work is now. Your personal transformation must fuel our collective liberation. Use your voice, find your coalition, and sustain your fight to ensure that every family has the right to live and raise their children in a truly safe and healthy world.

ABOUT THE AUTHOR

"My soul's work centers on creating moments where people's understanding is fundamentally shifted, empowering them with knowledge that creates lasting impact in their lives and communities."

Dr. DeShawn Taylor is a gynecologist, family planning specialist, gender-affirming care provider, associate clinical professor, and Reproductive Justice advocate. She advances reproductive healthcare access through direct services, education, training, advocacy, and leadership.

Dr. Taylor operates the Desert Star Health Justice Clinic in Phoenix, Arizona, under the umbrella of the nonprofit Desert Star Institute for Family Planning, which also leads coalition work, trains future abortion providers, and provides community education and programs that empower people from marginalized communities to exercise autonomy over their bodies and lives.

Throughout her career, Dr. Taylor has been the recipient of numerous awards:

- Recognized as a Trailblazer by the Maricopa County NAACP
- Honored as a Champion of Choice by the National Institute for Reproductive Health
- Awarded the Advocate of the Year Award from the Women's Foundation for the State of Arizona
- Received the Rashbaum Leadership Award from the Physicians for Reproductive Health

Dr. Taylor's mission is to equip advocate-minded individuals to speak about abortion effectively, organize around abortion and intersecting issues, and advance policies to improve access to care.

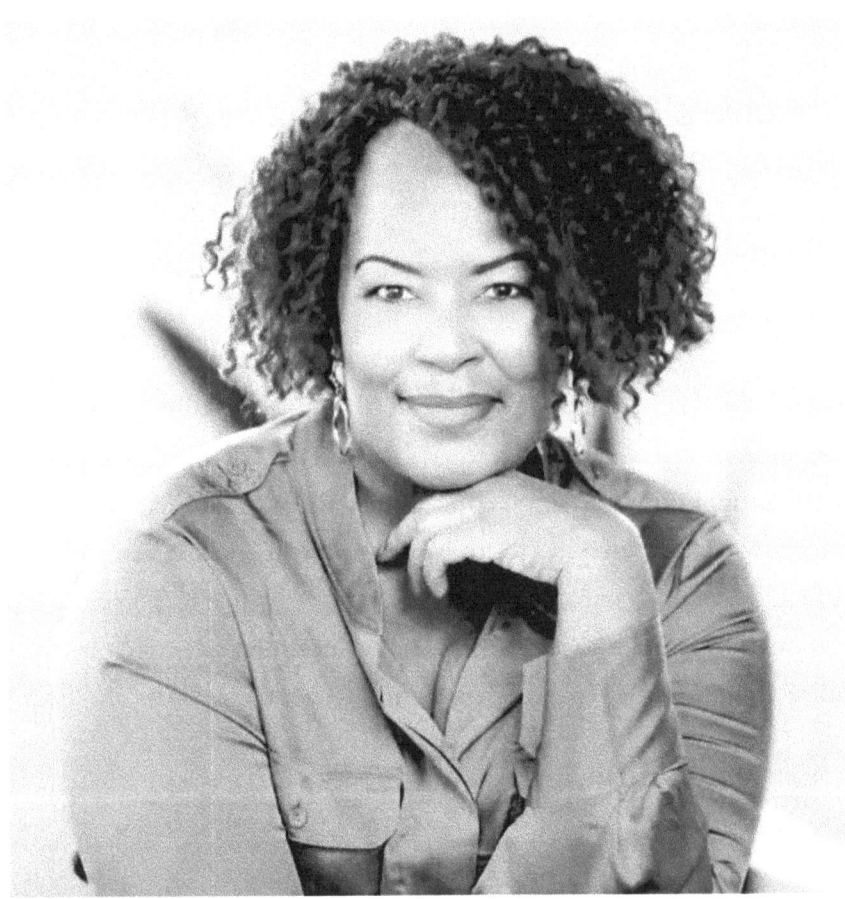

NOTES

Case Study: When Life Begins (and Ends): The Adriana Smith Story

1 Jeanine Santucci, "A Woman is Declared Brain Dead. A Georgia Law Forces Her to Carry Pregnancy, Report Says," *USA Today*, May 15, 2025, updated May 16, 2025, 6:25 a.m. ET, https://www.usatoday.com/story/news/nation/2025/05/15/georgia-abortion-law-braid-dead-life-support-pregnancy/83644831007/.

2 Miguel Legoas, "GoFundMe Set Up for Brain-Dead Pregnant Georgian. What We Know about Her Case," *Athens Banner-Herald*, May 21, 2025, https://www.onlineathens.com/story/news/2025/05/21/gofund-me-for-adriana-smith-of-georgia-brain-dead-and-pregnant/83767759007/

3 Sam Gringlas, "A Brain-Dead Woman's Pregnancy Raises Questions About Georgia's Abortion Law," *NPR*, May 21, 2025, 8:55 a.m. ET, https://www.npr.org/2025/05/21/nx-s1-5405542/a-brain-dead-womans-pregnancy-raises-questions-about-georgias-abortion-law.

4 Ibid.

5 Ibid.

6 Rachel Dobkin, "Family of Woman Who Carried Baby While Brain Dead Give Heartbreaking Update on Child: 'It's Not Getting Any Better Day by Day,' Adriana Smith's Mother Said of Her Grief

in a Recent Interview," *The Independent*, August 27, 2025, 18:51 EDT, https://www.the-independent.com/news/world/americas/adriana-smith-child-brain-dead-georgia-abortion-ban-b2815401.html.

7 Katha Pollitt, *Pro* (New York: Picador: 2014), 29.

8 For a detailed discussion of how different faith communities view when life begins, see my book, *Undue Burden* (Advantage Media: 2023).

9 April Newkirk, *Help Adriana's Family During This Heartbreaking Journey*, GoFundMe, accessed May 26, 2025, https://www.gofundme.com/f/help-adrianas-family-during-this-heartbreaking-journey.

10 American Civil Liberties Union of Georgia, "Reproductive Freedom," ACLU of Georgia, accessed May 26, 2025, https://www.acluga.org/en/issues/reproductive-freedom.

11 Becca Longmire, "Son of Georgia Woman Who Gave Birth While Brain Dead Is 'Making Progress' in the Hospital, Says Family," *People*, August 28, 2025, https://people.com/baby-of-georgia-woman-adriana-smith-who-gave-birth-brain-dead-making-progress-hospital-11799337.

Chapter 2: Moving Beyond "Choice"

12 Katha Pollitt, *Pro* (New York: Picador: 2014), 36-37.

13 Loretta Ross, "Understanding Reproductive Justice: Transforming the Pro-Choice Movement," *Off Our Backs*: 36. 5. 10.2307/20838711 (2006), https://www.researchgate.net/publication/259857714_Understanding_Reproductive_Justice_Transforming_the_Pro-Choice_Movement.

14 Kimala Price, "What is Reproductive Justice? How Women of Color Activists are Redefining the Pro-Choice Paradigm," *Meridians*, Vol 10 No2 (2011), 42-65. https://gws.illinois.edu/system/files/2022-05/WK%2013_Price_What%20is%20Reproductive%20Justice__0.pdf

15 Loretta Ross, "Understanding Reproductive Justice: Transforming the Pro-Choice Movement," *Off Our Backs*: 36. 14-19. 10.2307/20838711 (2006), https://www.researchgate.net/publication/259857714_Understanding_Reproductive_Justice_Transforming_the_Pro-Choice_Movement.

Chapter 3: How Reproductive Justice Touches Everything

16 See, Linda Villarosa, *Under the Skin: The Hidden Toll of Racism on American Lives and on the Health of Our Nation* (New York: Doubleday), pages 80-84 for a more detailed explanation of weathering and Geronimus' work.

Chapter 4: Connecting the Personal to the Political

17 Jamie R Daw et al. "Racial and Ethnic Disparities in Perinatal Insurance Coverage." *Obstetrics and gynecology* vol. 135,4 (2020): 917-924. doi:10.1097/AOG.0000000000003728, https://www.ncbi.nlm.nih.gov/pmc/articles/PMC7098441/.

18 Thomas E. Dobbs, State Health Officer of the Mississippi Department of health, et al., Petitioners, v. Jackson Women's Health Organization, et al., brief amicus curiae of Physicians for Reproductive Health, et al, 4, https://www.supremecourt.gov/DocketPDF/19/19-1392/192897/20210920113504270_210195a%20Amicus%20Brief%20for%20efiling.pdf

19 "What Is Stillbirth?" Centers for Disease Control, accessed Sept 30, 2022, https://www.cdc.gov/ncbddd/stillbirth/facts.html#:~:text=Stillbirth%20affects%20about%201%20in,stillborn%20in%20the%20United%20States.Perez

20 "Neonatal Death," March of Dimes, accessed Sept 30, 2022, https://www.marchofdimes.org/complications/neonatal-death.aspx#:~:text=Neonatal%20death%20happens%20in%20about,year%20in%20the%20United%20States.

21 "After Four Long Years in Prison, Adora Perez's Murder Charge for Stillbirth Is Dropped," National Advocates for Pregnant Women, Press Release, May 9, 2022, https://www.nationaladvocatesforpregnantwomen.org/adora-perez-case-dismissed/.

22 "Infant Mortality and African Americans," US Department of Health and Human Services, accessed Aug 1, 2022, https://minorityhealth.hhs.gov/omh/browse.aspx?lvl=4&lvlid=23#:~:text=Non%2DHispanic%20blacks%2FAfrican%20Americans,to%20non%2DHispanic%20white%20infants.

23 "Adolescent Sexual and Reproductive Health in the United States," Guttmacher Institute Fact Sheet, Sep 2019, https://www.guttmacher.org/fact-sheet/american-teens-sexual-and-reproductive-health.

Case Study: The Criminalization of Pregnancy Loss—The Brittany Watts Story

24 All details and quotations in this case study about Watt's pregnancy and arrest are taken from her first-hand account as told to Jericka Duncan, Rachel Bailey, and Hilary Cook, "Brittany Watts, Ohio Woman Charged with Felony After Miscarriage at Home, Describes Shock of Her Arrest," *CBS News*, updated October 21, 2024, https://www.cbsnews.com/news/brittany-watts-the-ohio-woman-charged-with-a-felony-after-a-miscarriage-talks-shock-of-her-arrest/.

25 I've adapted my four main principles from the twelve principles presented by Andrea J. Ritchie, Maria Thomas, and Fabián Fernández in their presentation, "Beyond Do No Harm," SisterSong Let's Talk About Sex Conference, Dallas, Texas, Aug 25-28. You can find more on Ritchie and Thomas's work at interruptingcriminalization.com.

26 Samantha Artiga, "Living in an Immigrant Family in America: How Fear and Toxic Stress are Affecting Daily Life, Well-Being, & Health," Kaiser Family Foundation, Dec 13, 2017, https://www.kff.org/racial-equity-and-health-policy/issue-brief/living-in-an-immigrant-family-in-america-how-fear-and-toxic-stress-are-affecting-daily-life-well-being-health/.

27 Nazish Dholakia, "Women's Incarceration Rates Are Skyrocketing. These Advocates Are Trying to Change That," Vera.org, May 17, 2021, https://www.vera.org/news/womens-voices/womens-incarceration-rates-are-skyrocketing.

Chapter 5: Faith and Abortion Care

28 Hovey G., "Abortion: A History," *Planned Parenthood Review*, 1985 Summer; 5(2):18-21. PMID: 12340403. https://pubmed.ncbi.nlm.nih.gov/12340403/.

29 Rachel K. Jones, "People of All Religions Use Birth Control and Have Abortions," Guttmacher Institute, October 2020, https://www.guttmacher.org/article/2020/10/people-all-religions-use-birth-control-and-have-abortions.

30 "U.S. Public Continues to Favor Legal Abortion, Oppose Overturning Roe v. Wade," Pew Research Center, Aug 29, 2019, https://www.pewresearch.org/politics/2019/08/29/u-s-public-continues-to-favor-legal-abortion-oppose-overturning-roe-v-wade/.

31 "Just the Facts: Catholic Perspectives on Sex, Gender, and Reproductive Health," Catholics for Choice, PDF, 4. https://www.catholicsforchoice.org/wp-content/uploads/2022/03/CatholicsForChoiceJustTheFacts.pdf.

32 "What We Believe: Abortion/Reproductive Choice Issues," Presbyterian Church (U.S.A.), accessed Sept 30, 2022, https://www.presbyterianmission.org/what-we-believe/social-issues/abortion-issues/.

33 "American Baptist Resolution Concerning Abortion and Ministry in the Local Church," ReligiousInstitute.org, accessed Sep 30, 2022, http://religiousinstitute.org/denom_statements/american-baptist-resolution-concerning-abortion-and-ministry-in-the-local-church/.

Chapter 6: Culture, Power, and the Fight for Inclusive Care

34 Caleb Smith, "New Survey Shows Abortion Bans' Unique and Chilling Impact on LGBTQI+ People," *Center for American Progress*, May 8, 2025, https://www.americanprogress.org/article/new-survey-shows-abortion-bans-unique-and-chilling-impact-on-lgbtqi-people/.

35 Ibid.

36 Alvin Powell, "The Problems with LGBTQ Health Care," *Harvard Gazette*, March 23, 2018, https://news.harvard.edu/gazette/story/2018/03/health-care-providers-need-better-understanding-of-lgbtq-patients-harvard-forum-says/.

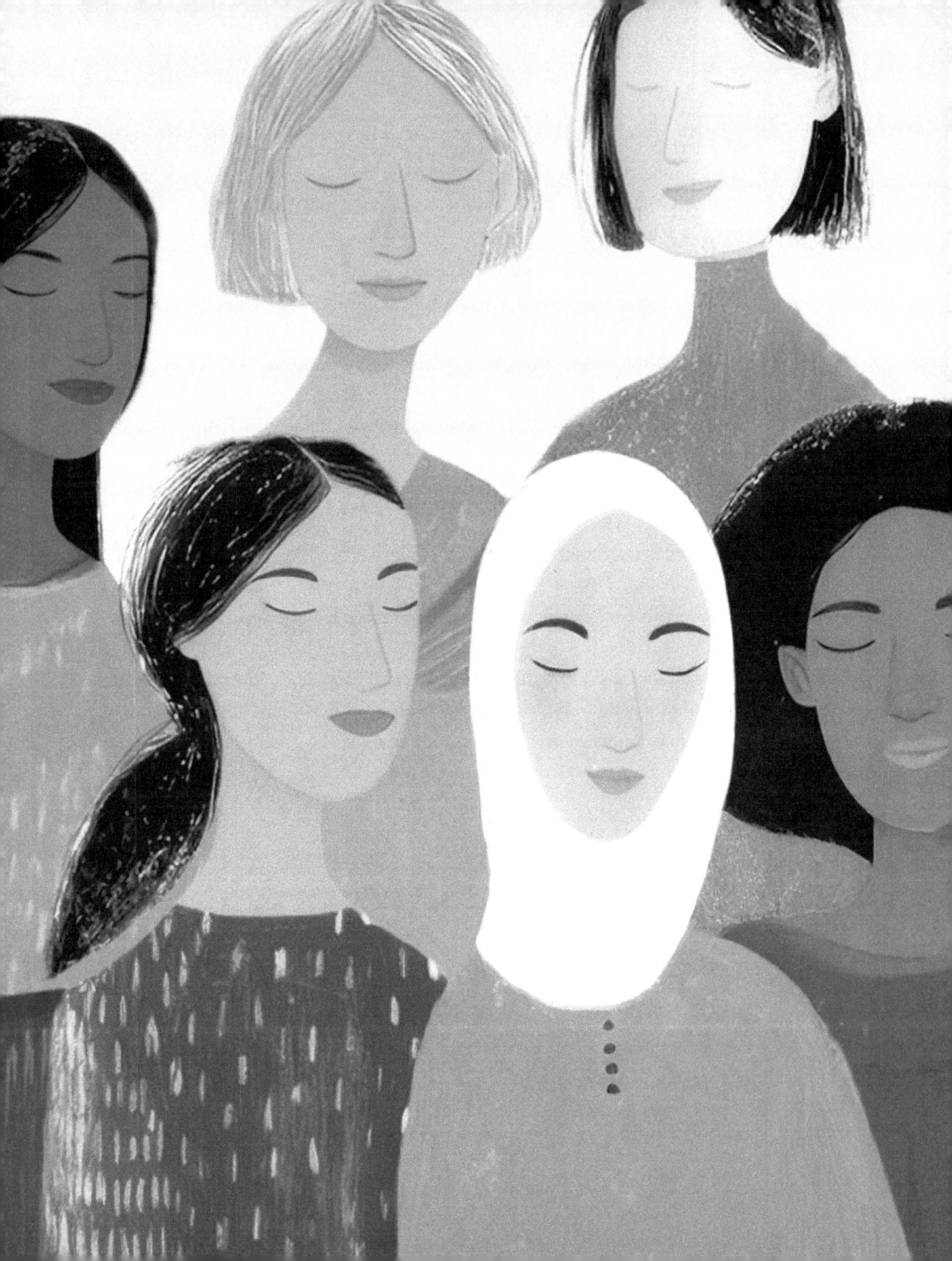

RESOURCES AND FURTHER READING

Resources

Reproductive Justice Organizations to follow and support that center people of color:

Desert Star Institute for Family Planning — A Black-led independent reproductive health and justice organization providing clinical care, professional training, and policy advocacy.
desertstarfp.org

Forward Together — A national multiracial organization advancing reproductive justice and family well-being through organizing, policy work, and cultural strategy.
forwardtogether.org

In Our Own Voice — A national organization dedicated to building power for Black women and girls across the reproductive justice movement.
blackrj.org

National Latina Institute for Reproductive Justice — A national organization advancing reproductive health and rights for Latinx communities through advocacy, leadership development, and community mobilization.
latinainstitute.org

SisterSong — A coalition of organizations led by women and people of color focused on amplifying the Reproductive Justice movement.
sistersong.net

URGE — A youth-driven organization organizing young people nationwide to advance Reproductive Justice through civic engagement and leadership development.
urge.org

Further Reading

Davis, Dána-Ain. *Reproductive Injustice: Racism, Pregnancy, and Premature Birth.* New York: NYU Press, 2019.

Fried, Marlene Gerber, and Loretta J. Ross. *Abortion and Reproductive Justice: An Essential Guide for Resistance.* First edition. Berkeley: University of California Press, 2025.

hooks, bell. *Feminist Theory: From Margin to Center.* Boston: South End Press, 1984.

Roberts, Dorothy E. *Killing the Black Body: Race, Reproduction, and the Meaning of Liberty.* New York: Pantheon Books, 1997.

Ross, Loretta J., and Rickie Solinger. *Reproductive Justice: An Introduction.* Oakland, CA: University of California Press, 2017.

Silliman, Jael Miriam, Marlene Gerber Fried, Loretta J. Ross, and Elena R. Gutiérrez. *Undivided Rights: Women of Color Organizing for Reproductive Justice.* Cambridge, MA: South End Press, 2004.

Srinivasan, Amia. *The Right to Sex: Feminism in the Twenty-First Century.* New York: Farrar, Straus and Giroux, 2021.

Taylor, DeShawn, MD. *Undue Burden: A Black Woman Physician on Being Christian and Pro-Abortion in the Reproductive Justice Movement.* New York: Advantage Media Group, 2023.

www.ingramcontent.com/pod-product-compliance
Lightning Source LLC
Chambersburg PA
CBHW080541030426

42337CB00024B/4812